P9-DTS-234

RENEWALS 691-4574

Psychotherapy—The Promised Land?

Psychiatric Outpatient Centers of America (POCA) is an organization comprising Psychiatric Clinics and Community Mental Health Centers in the United States, Canada, and Mexico. Founded in 1963, some of its many purposes have been to: disseminate information of importance to its clinic membership, offer consultative services to new and established agencies, organize forums for discussing mutual professional and administrative problems, make available group insurance plans for member clinics as well as other group benefits, publish lasting literature in the field and a newsletter covering current information relative to legislation, etc. POCA holds an annual spring meeting that provides much of the material presented in these volumes. Though special services of POCA are available only to member clinics, the annual meeting is open to all interested professionals and nonprofessionals.

For further information contact:

DR. MICHAEL DINOFF
POCA
Box 6142
University, Al. 35486

Psychotherapy—The Promised Land?

Edited by
MICHAEL DINOFF, Ph.D.
MILDRED ELLIOTT BERL, M.A.
ROBERT L. VOSBURG, M.D.

POCA Perspectives No. 6

WITHDRAWN
UTSA LIBRARIES

THE UNIVERSITY OF ALABAMA PRESS

University, Alabama

Library of Congress Cataloging in Publication Data
Main entry under title:

Psychotherapy—the promised land?

(POCA perspectives ; no. 6)
1. Psychotherapy. I. Dinoff, Michael.
II. Berl, Mildred E. III. Vosburg, Robert L.
IV. Series: Psychiatric Outpatient Centers of
America. POCA perspectives ; no. 6. [DNLM:
1. Community mental health services—Congresses.
2. Psychotherapy—Congresses. W1 P658 no. 6 /
WM420 P971p 1974-75]
RC480.5.P78   616.8'914   77-324
ISBN 0-8173-2730-4

Copyright © 1977 by
The University of Alabama Press
All rights reserved
Manufactured in the United States of America

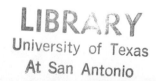
LIBRARY
University of Texas
At San Antonio

To
LEO KANNER, M.D.
Recipient, Fifth Annual Award,
Psychiatric Outpatient Centers of America*
for his work in the field of child or pediatric psychiatry

and

THEODORE LIDZ, M.D.
Recipient, Sixth Annual Award,
Psychiatric Outpatient Centers of America*
for his work in family research and therapy

*Previous recipients:
Gerald Caplan, M.D.
Rollo May, Ph.D.
Hon. William O. Douglas

Contributors

Hans J. Arndt, M.D., F.R.C.P. (C), Staff Psychiatrist, Humber Memorial Hospital, Toronto, Ontario.

Fern J. Azima, Ph.D., Associate Professor, Department of Psychiatry, McGill University, Montreal, Canada.

Bernard J. Bergen, Ph.D., Associate Professor of Psychiatry (Sociology), Dartmouth Medical School, Hanover, New Hampshire.

Mildred Elliott Berl, M.A., Psychologist, Director, Agnes Bruce Greig School and Center, Washington, D.C.

Michael Dinoff, Ph.D., Professor of Psychology and Director, Psychological Clinic, The University of Alabama, University, Alabama.

Matthew J. Friedman, M.D., Assistant Professor of Psychiatry, Dartmouth Medical School, Staff Psychiatrist, V.A. Hospital, White River Junction, Vermont.

Lewey O. Gilstrap, Jr., Cyberneticist, Private Consultant, Washington, D.C., President, Agnes Bruce Greig School and Center, Washington, D.C.

Judy Greer, O.T., Supervisor in Psychiatric Occupational Therapy, St. Michael's Hospital, Toronto, Ontario.

Etsuko Inselburg, M.A., M.S.W., Instructor in Clinical Psychiatry, Department of Psychiatry, Dartmouth Medical School.

Carolyn Kessler, Ph.D., Professor of Linguistics, Immaculate College of Washington, Washington, D.C.

Theodore Lidz, M.D., Professor of Psychiatry, Yale University School of Medicine, New Haven, Connecticut, and Career Investigator, National Institute of Mental Health.

Irving Markowitz, M.D., Psychiatrist, Family Service and Child Guidance Center, East Orange, New Jersey.

Connie E. Naitove, A.T.R., President of the New England Association of Art Therapists.

Phileo Nash, Ph.D., Professor of Anthropology, American University, Washington, D.C.

Luther D. Robinson, M.D., Sc.D., at the time of the conference, was superintendent of St. Elizabeth's Hospital, Washington, D.C., and is now associated with St. Elizabeth's.

William J. Stauble, M.D., C.M., F.R.C.P. (C), F.A.P.A., Psychiatrist-in-chief, St. Michael's Hospital, Toronto, Ontario.

Robert L. Vosburg, M.D., Psychiatrist, Dartmouth-Hitchcock Clinic, School of Medicine, Dartmouth College, Hanover, New Hampshire.

Contents

Foreword x

Preface to Part I: Communication and Creativity in
Psychotherapy
    Mildred Elliott Berl 2
Creative Arts Therapy
    Connie E. Naitove 3
Fingerpainting in Assessing Treatment
    Judy Greer, Hans J. Arndt, William J. Stauble 9
Rediscovering Tribalism
    Phileo Nash 17
Communication and the Deaf Patient
    Luther D. Robinson 25
Effective Communication in Adolescent Group Psychotherapy
    Fern J. Azima 31
The Machine as Diagnostician and Therapist
    Lewey O. Gilstrap, Jr. 43
The Impact of the Women's Liberation Movement on
Male Identity
    Robert L. Vosburg 53

Preface to Part II: Self, Salvation, and Psychotherapy
    Robert L. Vosburg 64
Which Self Does Psychotherapy Realize?
    Irving Markowitz 65
The Family and the Self
    Theodore Lidz 73
Self-Image in Pair Relationships
    Etsuko Inselburg 91
The Place of Drugs in Psychotherapy
    Matthew J. Friedman 101
Child Language and an Emerging Sense of Self
    Carolyn Kessler 111
Psychotherapy and the Dilemma of the Death and
Rebirth of the Self
    Bernard J. Bergen 125

Foreword

Each year The Association of Psychiatric Outpatient Centers of America, Inc. (POCA) publishes the papers of its annual convention. Because of the unique nature of the last two annual meetings, i.e., Washington 1974, and Boston 1975, it seemed wiser to publish them jointly since there were fewer formal papers. Of course the reduction in papers led to more interaction and dialogue. However, the result of combining the papers from these two meetings is that it is hard to generate a continuity of theme, and, harder yet, to title the volume.

The Washington meeting was devoted to "Creativity and Communication in Psychotherapy" while the Boston convention attended to the topic "Self, Salvation, and Psychotherapy." We have chosen to section this volume into a Part I (Washington) and a Part II (Boston). Both meetings focus upon the contemporary issues and dilemmas of the psychotherapist. It occurs to us that a title *Psychotherapy—The Promised Land?* might tie together the loosely woven themes of the two conferences.

As yet we do not know all we can or cannot do with psychotherapy. Each of us has gone through a period of our professional life when we wonder if we have oversold what we can do. Ultimately every psychotherapist comes to believe that the process of psychotherapy works. We see it every day in our clients and from the reports of our colleagues. Nevertheless there is so much more to learn.

MICHAEL DINOFF
MILDRED ELLIOTT BERL
ROBERT L. VOSBURG

Part I: Communication and Creativity in Psychotherapy

Preface to Part I: Communication and Creativity in Psychotherapy

MILDRED ELLIOTT BERL, M.A.

Several years ago, the writer visited one of the European countries as a consultant for children's services in a large hospital. The buildings were immaculate, the laboratories were impressive, and the clinical records were up-to-date and in good order. The children wandered aimlessly around in a courtyard during the day and slept in locked cubicles at night. There were no services other than feeding and clothing. Thirty kilometers away, near the top of a high mountain, I discovered another facility—a "kinderhaus," where there was much activity. Children were weaving, making nature prints, gathering fruit from a nearby orchard, and planning their evening meal in a group discussion. The number of children, their ages, and their clinical diagnoses were the same at the two institutions. The staff members at both places had the same professional designations. It seemed as though there were no communication across the valley that separated the two centers.

More recently, I met with outpatient clinic personnel at a POCA regional meeting concerned with services to the elderly. This meeting was in a state also divided by mountains and valleys with some creative programs that needed to be shared with those who were seeking ways and means of better service. Patients in one valley were separated from clinical services at a center across a river and up a mountain by a catchment area boundary.

Through our POCA conferences and regional workshops, we are striving to increase communication and to foster creativity. We recognize here the importance of developing communication with our patients through art, music, dance, drama, group activities, networks, and even machines. POCA's goal is better communication among those concerned with outpatient services in all geographical settings, in urban or rural areas, in Canada, Mexico, and the United States—or wherever we can reach across the valleys or over the mountains.

Creative Arts Therapy

Connie E. Naitove, A.T.R.

Creative Arts Therapy is based upon the premise that verbal and nonverbal behavior are related and that each of us has a nonverbal repertoire of symbolic expressions. In the therapeutic application of the arts, aesthetics are irrelevant. The essential issue is what the client finds out about himself through the use of art forms. By eliminating aesthetics, the stigma of failure is removed. This vital aspect can be reinforced by the use of uncommon or unfamiliar media and techniques, such as woodshavings and mime. The issues of talent and skill, which frustrate so many of us, are avoided and hesitancy and inhibition are readily overcome. Further, as an individual becomes cognizant of his own repertoire of creative art expression, he gains a sense of identity. Such an awareness frequently leads to the confidence necessary to cope with other areas where "risk" of failure has been the deterrent.

Most of the creative arts are recognized as basic forms of communication. However, the potential for use of these modes of expression in therapy is not so well appreciated. This lack of appreciation, in part, is owing to the tendency to equate creative expression with talent. As most of us are convinced that we have no talent, the Arts Therapist is continually being confronted by such statements as: "I can't draw a straight line; I have two left feet, a tin ear," or "I'm all thumbs!" It must be stressed that talent is not the limiting factor; rather, it is the inability to appreciate and utilize the artistic experiences that are common to all of us. We have lost sight of the components of color, form, texture, spacial relationships, sound, and rhythm that fill our environment. For those of you who feel you have no sense of rhythm it can be pointed out that en utero you existed in a point/counterpoint environment of two heartbeats. We all move to the natural rhythms or our breathing. Thus no one alive lacks a sense of rhythm. Similarly, anyone with the powers of speech can sing. It is instinctive, even in speech, for the voice to go up and down. If you write numbers and letters, you are drawing. If you doodle, you draw. Anyone who bakes bread or reads braille can sculpt. Anyone taking notes at the meeting is a potential artist. Creative Arts Therapy reawakens sensory awareness. It reminds us that sound is meant to be listened to and that movement is as inherent in us as color is in our environment; it utilizes this awareness to create symbolic expressions.

The Arts provide a natural outlet for nonverbal symbolic expression. Through the Arts, we can interrelate common symbolic references in speech, form, and gesture. One grasps my meaning immediately when I refer to our "colorful" speech: eg., feeling "blue," a "blue joke" or a "blue law." Our language is also dynamically symbolic, as when we are "down," "high," or simply a "pushover." Many of our words are applicable equally to all the arts. Up, down, long, short, heavy, light, strong, weak, can be applied appropriately to music, movement, drawing, or architecture; the application of these terms facilitates communication across the mythical barriers to using the Arts in therapy.

Eliciting and enhancing the clients' awareness of his own, often unique symbolic repertoire, gives a sense of identity, of self-image, as well as a problem-identifying/solving set of tools. Rather than one cookbook of symbolic expressions, applicable across the board, it should be emphasized that each individual has his own personal repertoire of which he is the only valid translator. Thus, each client is advised at the outset that aesthetics are irrelevant, that the purpose of these activities is increased self-awareness, and that the therapist is merely the facilitator, while the client remains the sole responsible interpreter of what is expressed.

Ours is a short-term diagnostic hospital and our techniques have been used in one-to-one and group therapy sessions with equal success. These techniques have been designed for groups of mixed ages (often varying from 13 to 78 years of age) and are adaptable for use with the handicapped and infirmed. Primarily we use art, movement, mime, and music, singly or in combination, with individuals from varying social, economic, and educational backgrounds. We begin our sessions with a warm-up activity designed to facilitate body movement, release physical and emotional tensions, and acquaint the group with each other, the therapist, and the media. We use exercises that progress from the use of digits to involvement of the whole extremity to total body awareness, involving large and small muscle activity. In the process of these activities, an awareness of the individual gesture and its relationship to the environment, both natural and social, is emphasized. We then proceed to a core activity that involves one or more of the arts. Finally the session concludes with a discussion of reactions to the entire activity.

Although acting primarily as the initiator of creative expression, the therapist must also be alert for idiosyncratic patterns, observing correlations and discrepancies between verbalizations, movements, mime, and the uses of space, color, and line. The client's drawings may be loose while his movements constrained, his speech colorful, his pictures not. The therapist should be sensitive and factual in pointing out these discrepancies to the client.

Art media are selected to allow for rapid, unrestricted movements, rather than those which support compulsive behaviors. Marking pens are favored over erasable media such as pencil, as the latter tends to severely limit productivity. The warm-up activity in art is the "scribble": a large-muscle activity that is valuable for expanding creativity. Both subjective and projective techniques can be superimposed upon it and it invariably brings a laugh.

It is our purpose in using mime to make the client aware that, while he cannot escape his body, he neither lives nor moves in a vacuum. We point out that each act is a phrase, a personal communication, and that gagged or oversimplified acting is either inappropriate or inadequate to such communication. The client is simultaneously encouraged to correlate this behavior to other social encounters.

Music is used as a facilitator of all activities as well as a dictionary of pattern and rhythm. The therapist will point out that the voice of an instrument can be correlated to color, texture, or volume and that the rhythms of music and movement can be depicted simply by the number and repetitions of linear movements. The progression can be reversed; the linear movements in a yarn picture, for example, can be correlated to physical movement and the use of space. Rhythm is, after all, merely the figure/ground relationship encountered in a time dimension, while dance or movement is merely time in a physical dimension.

An example of a simple progression used begins with a warm-up activity in which large-muscle groups are loosened and stretched in rhythmic accompaniment to music. Carrying this large-muscle activity over to another media, we would all then do a scribble. It might be suggested that we seek out forms suggested by the lines, or add colors to it, for self, likes, or dislikes, etc. Or we might create a new pattern for how we feel right now, and, later move physically according to the patterns created. This last progression frequently enhances verbalizations such as, "I always seem to go around in circles; I don't seem to get anywhere." The client making such a statement is encouraged to enact his drawing physically to see if he cannot alter this pattern. Drawing what has transpired physically and emotionally, using line and color, often brings out more than simple verbalizations, and the client becomes aware that he has options to avoid or alter undesired patterns of behavior.

On another occasion, we might begin by tossing a beanbag back and forth, getting to know each others' names, and then progressing to a partner activity in mime, such as mirroring the cleaning of a glass door. This social and physical interaction is carried a step further in nonverbal communication by having one partner mime the painting of a large mural while the other enacts his exact mirror image. This exercise completed, both then proceed to different sheets of paper, away from each other, in an attempt to depict the mural just created in mime. We might then proceed to mimed role-enactments, such as parent/child relationships or abstract relationships, such as point/counterpoint, purple and yellow, dualities and opposites.

Some sessions proceed from simple eye contact, meeting-rejecting-reconciling-parting mime, to relationships of contest and trust (using shoulder-to-shoulder, hip-to-hip contests and mutual weight balancing and support) among partners. Drawing how these activities made one feel enhances verbalization and social adjustments and also stresses social and body awareness.

Progressions involving trust may begin on the floor, relaxing with eyes closed; exploring one's face, both relaxed and grimacing as well as how one would like others to see us. The next sequence can have one partner leading the other, who has his eyes closed, over an imaginary terrain. It is important not only to have partners reverse roles of dependence and responsibility but also to change partners, in order to discourage over-reliance on one individual. We always follow such activity with drawings relating to how one felt in each of the roles experienced.

In another session, the sequence might progress from unit awareness, to moving as if one were a machine, to drawing oneself as a machine; from moving as an animal, to drawing oneself as an animal. These machines or animals might then be cut out and added to a mural on a theme, such as Noah's ark, with options to move them about as desired, while the reasons and reactions are discussed with the group. Mural themes may be predetermined by the therapist or left to the client or group to determine, but themes can usually be found that relate to the clients' self-image and where they are at the moment.

Other techniques which we have found useful and popular involve collage: using photos of clients, words, and magazine photos, torn and cut to represent "rough" or simple emotional responses, based upon themes of past-present-future progressions, or dualities such as male/female, likes and dislikes. The relationships depicted are discussed, enacted, and, finally, if desired, altered. An example might be a depiction of important members of a given community (family, group, or residential community) that may illuminate feelings of isolation. A client with such demonstrable feelings might be asked if or how he might like to overcome this feeling and thus alter his relationship with others. He might then draw a line from himself to and around another individual depicted on the mural. Having done so, he would be asked if he would like actually to embrace the other or a surrogate, and if not, why not, and if so, how it felt to have taken this action. Such techniques have proved educative to both the individual and the group. Situational enactment using client-created clay or cut-out cardboard figures is another technique that enables clients to explore social relationships and self-image without threat and has proved very satisfying.

While it is likely that the therapist will predetermine the media combination of a given session, it is helpful to have several activity progressions in mind before beginning any Creative Arts session. It is wise for the therapist to remain flexible and be on the ready to "play it by ear" according to immediate client needs. On occasion we have found that the group merely wanted to do a variety of movements to music; once we spent twenty minutes "skating" about the room! On another occasion, a collage mural occupied the group for the entire hour and a half allotted for these workshops, and still the clients were unwilling to stop.

It has been our experience that, whereas thirty minutes to an hour may be the maximum tolerance for a dynamic arts activity, clients prefer an hour to ninety minutes for graphic or plastic arts. We have concluded that ninety minutes is a minimum for an interrelated Creative Arts experience, and that two hours is the maximum tolerance without exhausting the clients' as well as the therapists' physical and emotional reserves. We have little difficulty sustaining attendance and interest for this period as the progressions are rapid and client-oriented.

There are many reports in the literature of the therapeutic application of art, mime, movement, music, poetry, drama, and even horticulture. The use of creative expression by communities to overcome apathy, reduce delinquency and vandalism, improve individuals physically and socially, and increase productivity has been well documented. In our own experience, students, teachers, the indigent and incarcerated of all ages have gained confidence, motivation, and an improved awareness of self and body image, as well as an increased sense of reality. Indeed, Freud, himself, noted that, "There is, in fact, a way from fantasy back to reality, and that is—ART!" (Freud: 23rd Introductory Lecture).

BIBLIOGRAPHY

American Horticulturist. Vol. 52, No. 3, p. 19–25.

Ashton-Warner, Sylvia. *Teacher*. Simon & Schuster, 1963.

Brandreth, Gyles. *Created in Captivity*. Hodder & Stoughton, Ltd., 1972.

Harris, Jay and Joseph, Cliff. *Murals of the Mind*. International University Press, Inc., 1973.

Kock, Kenneth. *Wishes, Lies and Dreams*. Vantage Books, 1970.

Kramer, Edith. *Art as Therapy with Children*. New York: Schoken Books, 1971.

Kris, Ernst. *Psychoanalytic Explorations in Art*. London, 1953.

North, Marion. *An Introduction to Movement Study and Teaching*. Macdonald & Evans, Ltd.

Sachs, Hanns. *The Creative Unconscious*. 1942.

Slade, Peter. *Child Drama*. University of London Press. 1955.

Wethered, Audrey G. *Drama and Movement in Therapy*. Macdonald & Evans, Ltd.

Fingerpainting
in Assessing Treatment

Judy Greer, O.T.

Hans J. Arndt, M.D., F.R.C.P. (C)

William J. Stauble, M.D.,

C.M., F.R.C.P. (C), F.A.P.A.

Ours is a case presentation with several interesting twists: first, a rather interesting patient; second, the use of the Lehmann Scales in evaluating a series of fingerpainting; and third, the use of large amounts of chlorpromazine in the treatment of psychosis.

The patient was a 33-year-old married woman with three children. She had been in a large psychiatric hospital for five months in a regressive psychotic state, and there was some doubt as to whether she would ever be able to return to her family. She had two brief psychiatric hospitalizations following the delivery of her last child. The hope was that with highly concentrated treatment, she would have a slight chance of recovery. The initial impression on admission to our inpatient unit was that the lady was suffering from a severe psychotic illness. Soon after admission, referrals were made to the Psychology Department for a full assessment, to the Social Work Department for a family assessment, and to the Occupational Therapy Department for vocational and projective evaluation. Her medication was a modest 100 mg. thioridazine. She presented herself on admission with a very flat affect and had no insight at all, but there was no sign of thought disorder. After a week, paranoid delusions began to appear, and a MMPI test done in the Psychology Department indicated that she was a well-guarded, overcontrolled schizophrenic.

That weekend she went home on a two-day pass and returned in a regressed state, out of touch, unaware of others around her, burning herself with cigarettes. Her medications were increased 600 mg. chlorpromazine and one week later were as high as 1000 mg. It was decided, at the time of increasingly high dosage of medication, that a series of fingerpainting would be helpful to give an objective evaluation of the effects of medication since this dosage was relatively high. The patient was too regressed to continue with psychological testing.

The patient was suspected of not actually taking her medication in tablet form and her fingerpaintings were showing deterioration in the evaluating scales. She was switched to liquid-form medication and was raised to 1250 mg. chlorpromazine. There was still some difficulty in convincing her to accept the medications. On this amount, the patient appeared a little drowsy, but the drowsiness disappeared in three days. A slight degree of improvement was noted clinically, as well as in the fingerpaintings. After her medications were raised to 2000 mg. then to 2500 mg. chlorpromazine, no further clinical regression was noted and her fingerpaintings were becoming more organized.

She had enough energy during an afternoon outing with patients to a park to join in a game of baseball and hit seven home runs. While her personal hygiene had been very poor, there was now a change. The makeup was now well applied to her face without the smearing that had previously appeared. Her social skills were still very limited. After two months in hospital, she began to have regular weekend passes with her family, which after the first week went quite well. Her positive feelings about these times emerged in the paintings. A mother hen and her chicks, her dog and cat, and a nature scene she remembered from a week in the country. She was now taking her medications by tablet even when out of hospital, but a close eye was kept on the fingerpaintings in order that any regression could be noticed quickly. After 3½ months of inpatient hospitalization, she was discharged to Day Care with the fingerpaintings to be continued weekly. Her medications were increased to 3000 mg. to prevent a possible regression caused by the stress of discharge. This increase meant that she had to take 15 pills daily, 3 pills five times. The plan was to keep her on high medications for an extended period of time and gradually wean her away from hospital. She did well on full day care, although she was late every day and her social skills showed little change. Slight fluctuations in her hold on reality and in her personal hygiene were observed. One month later, her attendance was reduced to Day Care three times a week. There was slight regression with manipulative behavior, but this improved with talks about quicker discharge from Day

Care Treatment if she would cooperate with the treatment plan. The patient by this time was very keen to get back to her family. She was preoccupied with moving to a new house and enthusiastic about decorating. For the last two months of her treatment, she was only to attend twice, and later, once a week.

The happy ending to our story was that at our last contact, the patient was doing well at home. She had taken an office job and become active in church affairs in her community, all on 3000 mg. of chlorpromazine.

The Lehmann Scale

We chose the Lehmann Scales to evaluate the fingerpaintings because they are well documented, objective, and easy to use. They stress the formal aspect of production and provide a basis on which to make quantitative and qualitative comparisons. To obtain useful information, it is not so necessary to make detailed observations during production or to question the patient about interpretation of his painting.

The four categories in this method of rating are: energy output, contact with reality, affective range, and clarity.

Energy output is determined by the number of strokes, the pressure used, and the surface covered, i.e., quarter page, half page, full page. This scale should be an indication of how much energy the patient is putting into his daily routine.

Contact with reality is measured by the degree of realism in the painting. Descriptions of work in this category range from indefinable, bizarre, meaningless repetition, symbolism, abstract design, landscape, up to very detailed representations of objects and plants. From this scale we get an idea of how firm a hold on reality the patient has at the time of production.

Affective range rating is arrived at by adding values assigned to colors which the patient uses in the production. The method of assigning values to colors has been the subject of a great deal of controversy. Lehmann's method is quite simple and he feels it works well for the purposes of his scales. The colors, yellow and red, are thought of as warm, outgoing euphoric colors, while blue and green are thought to be cold subdued colors. Black and brown are thought to be somber colors, expressive of a depressed mood. Therefore, red and yellow are assigned a value of three, blue and green are valued at two, and black and brown are valued at one. Long and Dellis (1961) in their critique of the scales put forward the comment that the amount of area covered by a color is an important dimension of affectivity not acknowledged in these scales.

Clarity of the production is rated according to distinctiveness of line, separation of colors, clarity of design, and neatness of execution. Description of the productions for rating goes as follows: smearing and confusion, hazy, fairly distinct, up to meticulous. Lehmann says that it is the improvement in clarity that most reliably indicates improvement in a person's psychiatric condition.

The system of scoring is fairly simple. Each of the categories just mentioned has a maximum of 12 points and a minimum of 0. The scales are arranged so that the optimum or norm rating is at 8. Scores above and below the norm are seen as deviations representing lack of or excess of qualities assessed in the categories. In a study by Lehmann and Risquez (1953) findings were that nonpsychotics scored higher than other diagnostic groups in all four categories. The organic psychosis group was the lowest with the depressives a close second on the affective range scale, while the highest score was taken by the manic group. Manic patients also scored highest on the energy output scale with organic psychoses and depressives at the bottom. Organics scored lowest on the contact with reality scale with the schizophrenics also scoring low. In general, it should be noted that the areas of clarity and contact with reality seem to show almost equal deterioration in most severe mental disturbances, especially in the functional psychoses.

Over a period of six months the patient had done a series of 25 paintings. As the treatment went along, we were able to evaluate improvement or deterioration in her condition, and we could correlate changes with events in her environment, changes in medication, etc. This evaluation was especially important, since she was unreliable about taking the prescribed medication. As the goal of treatment was to move her back to the community, the patient was away from the hospital and the observers for increasingly longer periods of time. An objective evaluation of her condition by means of the rating scales coupled with clinical observation helped to indicate whether she was taking her medications while outside the hospital. The best indicator of readiness to return to her family was the consistency of the fingerpaintings during the last few months of treatment. Also, the fact that the content of the pictures changed from fantasy figures and symbols to representations of her environment showed an increased meaningfulness in her life outside the hospital.

Energy Output Graph. The first painting was rated very high. The whole page was covered with many directions of strokes, showing much activity. The first low rating at painting #5, occurred during the time the patient was suspected of not taking her medications. The next low rating occurred at picture #8, when there was a regression during Day Care. The patient was seclusive and forgetful of routines and medications. The day she painted, she had brought her daughter along for the day. Highs at paintings #18 and #19 occurred during the time Day Care was cut to three days a week.

Affective Range Graph. This graph shows less degree of variation from beginning to end of treatment. The high scores at paintings #18 and #21 correspond to the switch to less frequent Day Care and thoughts about the Christmas season. Her affect, which was initially flat, showed little change during treatment. Toward the end of hospitalization, the patient smiled and laughed more frequently, but interpersonal relationships remained on a superficial level.

Contact with Reality. This score we watched with the most interest. It has very wide fluctuations during early hospitalization, but during Day Care it becomes more consistent. The lower scores occurred after a very upsetting weekend at home (#1), before the medication was switched from tablet to liquid form (#6), and at the time of her first full weekend pass (#8). In the content of the paintings, the subject of the first few pictures contained symbols, whereas the last pictures showed interest in her environment and an increased ability to represent it realistically.

Clarity Scale. Low ratings at paintings #1 and #6 again correspond to those events previously mentioned. The interesting parallel is the improvement in clarity of her fingerpainting with the neatness of her makeup.

Combined Scale. This scale is arrived at by averaging the four scores for each of the paintings to give a general idea of the patient's psychiatric condition.

Conclusions

This study is obviously based on just one patient, and our presentation describes only one way of following a patient's progress in treatment. Objectivity is very difficult to attain in evaluating treatment, and hopefully, the use of the Lehmann Scales helped us to gain an increased measure of objectivity in the treatment of our patient. This technique seems applicable in the treatment of many patients. In southern Ontario, we have many ethnic communities in rural areas and in the cities, and it is not uncommon for patients referred to us to be nonfluent in English. A technique such as this one, could provide quite useful information about the patient's response to treatment when he cannot report verbally. In rural areas, a fingerpainting series could provide an objective and convenient method of follow-up. Many patients feel more comfortable with activity than with verbal communications; perhaps more use could be made of graphic productions in following these patients. In the case of patients lacking in awareness of the extent of their illness, a series of productions can serve to educate and perhaps prevent a recurrence of severe psychiatric illness.

Fingerpainting is a fascinating and imaginative medium with many applications.

The authors gratefully acknowledge the encouragement and assistance of Dr. Josif Divic, St. Michael's Hospital, Toronto, Ontario, Canada.

BIBLIOGRAPHY

Adamson, J., and Jackson, A. Relationships of Picture Content and Patients Age Diagnosis for Colour Choice. *American Journal of Occupational Therapy,* vol. 27, no. 1, 1973.

Anastasi, A., and Foley, J. P., Jr. Survey of the Literature on Artistic Behaviour in the Abnormal; 1 Historical and Theoretical Background. *Journal General Psychology,* 25: 111, 1941.

Azima, H., and Azima, E. Outline of a Dynamic Theory of Occupational Therapy. *American Journal of Occupational Therapy,* vol. 13, 1959.

Bendroth, S., and Southan, M. Objective Evaluation of Projective Material. *American Journal Occupational Therapy,* vol. 27, no. 2, 1973.

Brown, Walter L. *Introduction to Psycho-Oconography; The Interpretation and Use of Schizophrenic Art in Psycho-Therapy.* New Jersey: Schering Corporation, 1967.

Dorken, Herbert. The Reliability and Validity of Spontaneous Fingerpaintings. *Journal of Projective Techniques,* vol. 18, 1954.

Lawn, E. C., and Kane, C. P. Psychological Symbols as Communication Media. *American Journal of Occupational Therapy,* vol. 27, no. 1, 1973.

Lehmann, H. E. and Risquez, F. A. The Use of Fingerpaintings in the Clinical Evaluation of Psychotic Conditions; A Quantitative and Qualitative Approach. *Journal of Mental Science,* vol. 99, no. 417, 1953.

Long, I. Alan, and Dellis, Nicholas, P. Relationships Between the Fingerpainting and Overt Behaviour of Schizophrenics. *Journal of Projective Techniques,* 25, no. 2, 1961.

Naumberg, M. *Schizophrenic Art: Its Meaning in Psychotherapy,* New York: Grune and Stratton, 1950.

Rediscovering Tribalism

Phileo Nash, Ph.D.

As the first warm days of spring come to our college campuses this year, our libraries are not on fire. Presidents (college presidents, that is) work undisturbed in their offices and look out their windows and do not see a mob preparing a confrontation, only an occasional streaker.

Around the universities enrollments are declining at the same time that the draft ends. Campus posters still announce meetings on abortion or to hear George McGovern; but almost as many announce the presence of gurus, or meetings to discuss Zen or astral projection, or to learn yoga. In my own classes, the most popular works are no longer the Castaneda tetralogy, but books about how to get the mind to leave the body and travel to more interesting places.

So the young again baffle and mystify their elders. In my youth our professors felt that we were passive and uninterested in public affairs. Later generations troubled their elders because they were *too* much interested in public affairs. And now that things are more settled, not just on campuses but elsewhere, we find our cherished trust in rationality, mind-body unity, and the recourse to the ultimate metabolism unsettling—not the young but ourselves—the old, staid, and conventional.

So, I propose to explore briefly with you the phenomenon. It goes beyond ESP, Eastern philosophy, and transcendentalism. It goes to the good earth, to communal living, to nonmaterialism and the creation of a youth world, which is apart from adult participation and the values of the world of work. I am calling this phenomenon "tribalism," and I suggest that the search for it and the effort to realize it represents a discovery effort special to youth but fully the equivalent of such efforts as the discovery of new worlds or the exploration of space.

Any self-respecting social movement must have an identifying symbol that becomes a signal to the self and to others that there is a group with a boundary. Those who respond to the signal affirmatively reinforce the group identity by belonging; those who do not, reinforce it by not belonging. The primary signal is attire or the uniform of casualness. From the top down, much hair, steel-rimmed granny glasses, and clothes from the Goodwill. From the inside out, nothing that would indicate subservience to the merchandizing world.

But it would be a mistake to think that this attire is merely a way of dressing. With the dress goes a world view that we might call the "the good earth" syndrome. Natural foods, the ecology movement, and zero population growth are as much a part of this view as interest in Eastern religion. Such views are nonestablishment in their rejection of materialism, but even more in their unwillingness to accept the premise that nature can be managed, and that such management ("conservation") is good in and of itself. Nature, in this world view, is something to be harmonized with, not to be managed.

The college campus may be the apparent home of the movement but it is not a natural home for this group, or for that matter, for any group of young adults. No, the natural home for these young people is the commune. Washington, like many other cities across the country (and many rural centers), is dotted with old, nondescript unwanted dwellings that are available for little cost. Occupying these buildings are groups of young people who are determined to live nonmaterialistically, nonexploitively, and noncompetitively. Many of them are succeeding in the sense that they have been in existence for several years, and that their members pool resources, and share jobs, incomes, and windfalls.

It does not necessarily follow that the individual members of the commune are the same through long periods of time. Indeed, it is not essential to the philosophy of the movement that this kind of structural permanence should exist.

A tolerant attitude toward the use of drugs characterizes the public utterances of those who speak for the communes. At the same time the possibility of losing the premises if drugs are found has led to strict house rules on possession. Sexual liaisons come and go with relative ease, but if the investigations so far reported are reliable, pairings of this kind are less frequent and more stable than the stereotype suggests.

So much for the skeleton of this sub-culture. The anthropologist wants to know much more. Research is scanty and one has to rely on anecdotal reports. What is the class origin of the commune members? To what extent are they truly self-sufficient in dollars? Have they truly avoided the meaner aspects of the work ethic? What are the ratios of males to females? Of older and younger? What are the child-rearing practices in actuality as well as in the ideal? How are decisions arrived at? Last but not least, what justification (if any) do I have for calling this subset of behaviors "tribal?"

We are not completely devoid of data. Dr. John Bennett of Washington University, St. Louis, studied a wide variety of communities and prepared a report for a symposium held in Tucson, Arizona, a few years ago. Several films that portray life in communes, both urban and rural, and with alternate family constellations have been produced in recent years. No new configuration appears in America without polltakers sampling opinion within it and about it.

Generally speaking, the following things seem to be true of the communes:

(1) There is a continuous striving toward consensus government. By this term I mean that decisions affecting the commune are characteristically made (or it is felt that they should be made) by discussion ending in unanimity. Moreover, this type of government is felt to be the polar opposite of representative government with its brief discussion, formal votes, and majority-minority polarization.

(2) The members of the commune movement are almost exclusively of middle-class origin. Neither the very rich nor the very poor are attracted by communal living; the ethnic, racial, and religious minorities are conspicuously absent. Thus, Appalachian whites, blacks, and Spanish-speaking, to name just a few, are not represented in the newspaper stories I have seen. And, in the New Mexico communes, it is clear that there is open hostility on the part of the rural Spanish-speaking community, which has been on the land for two hundred years, to its commune neighbors who are, to a degree, imitating their life-style.

(3) A substantial degree of self-sufficiency has been achieved by hard work, resourcefulness, and ingenuity. Thus, by raising vegetables in the rural communes and by finding service occupations in the urban communes, the members have been able to avoid substantially the world of money and interest, loans and mortgages, taxes and forfeitures.

But it would also seem that these resources are supplemented in many cases by substantial remittances, gifts, loans, and allowances from middle-class and upper middle-class parents who cannot control, but who will not abandon the effort to regulate their children's lives, and find cash transmission the only acceptable medium of communication.

(4) Children are a part of the life of the communes. Very little information is available on actual child-rearing practices, and even less on the effects of communal living on personality formation. In this respect a golden opportunity to compare style and practices between the loosely structured communes and the highly structured *kibbutzim* is being lost.

There is a whole literature on the latter but almost no information on the former. The scanty information leads tentatively to the initial hypothesis that the commune pattern is to treat even the youngest children as miniature adults. They are, of course, taken everywhere the parent or parents go; they participate, at first passively, later actively, in such household chores as food preparation and in the endless discussions that accompany consensus decision. They are part and parcel of governance from an early age.

Education is again an unknown. The parents have a wholly predictable and understandable reluctance to expose children of the commune to the hazards of public school education if the environment is already hostile. Besides, the commune philosophy tends to support de-schooling, so a good deal of non-schooled education is going on in the communes and in free schools.

All these areas are endlessly fascinating but generate many more questions than answers. Is tribalism a fantasy of mine, or is it shared by others? I have been talking largely about American communes, specifically, those in the United States. To our young people "tribal" is more or less synonymous with "American Indian," especially with North American Indians north of Mexico. We can remove from consideration for present discussion purposes the highly organized tribes of Africa with elaborate chieftainships, hereditary rulers, and traditional courts of justice.

The American Indian bands, tribes, and pueblos with which the young people of today have become acquainted in person, or in anthropology courses, do, in fact conform rather well to the life-style idealized in the philosophy of the communes. The feeling of oneness with nature and the ideal of harmony with all living things are very much a part of the religion and world view of many American Indians. The conditions of crowded poverty that are common on most of the reservations may mock this world view, but the belief is there nevertheless. It is strong enough to account for the persistence of Indian culture in the face of unimaginable onslaughts by government, settlers, missionaries, and—I do not over-look my own profession—anthropologists.

I can also assure you that government by consensus was and still is the way of decision-making by many American Indian tribes. To be sure, it is often accompanied by a good deal of formal authority. The New Mexico pueblos, for example, are governed by traditional leaders who occupy their positions by a combination of right-by-descent and position in sacred societies. Under ordinary conditions they do not surface and by consensus their identity and exercise of authority is kept a private matter, especially from representatives of non-Indian governments.

This privacy has been true since the conquest in the sixteenth century, with its accompaniment of forced labor and religious conversion. The secretive organization of the rebellion of 1680 is the prototype of all matters that need not concern non-Indians, even non-Pueblo Indians. It is said that within this secret theocracy all decisions are arrived at by discussion and the establishment of a consensus. In matters where pueblo and the Federal government are concerned, there are two kinds of governance. If the federal government is intruding upon an area of exclusively pueblo concern (such as the entry of electricity within the old village) one can meet formally with the council but not much will happen. On the other hand, if the issue is properly one of external affairs, such as the Pueblo's share of water rights in the water conservancy district, there is no difficulty in meeting with the Council, where all members adopt the previously arrived at position.

In matters of child-rearing and education, the congruence between American Indian "tribal" and communal philosophy and practice is equally clear. The combination of permissiveness with expectations of internal control, unaccompanied by procedures for acquiring it and quick anger when it is not automatically present, is a characteristic of American middle-class behavior. It is one of the many things against which the youth culture is rebelling. In the traditional American Indian societies, even in the midst of substantial family breakdown and under conditions of severe deprivation, it is possible to see a very smooth relationship of kindness, protectiveness, and respect between parents and children. No one can spend time with a Hopi family, for example, without being aware of the continuous watchfulness over small children, unaccompanied by admonitions, nagging, or physical harassment. By

the same token it is the Hopis who have retained to the utmost their traditional culture, yet, who opened negotiations with the government of
the United States with a delegation requesting educational services.
Today, they still have a high rate of school attendance and a keen interest in the best of modern education.

So, in matters of their relationship to the environment, governance,
and schooling, the young people of today have a legitimate model in
certain aspects of the American Indian cultures of both the past and the
present.

This paradox is not a novelty as far as American cultural history is
concerned. The colonization of America coincided with two great ethical
and philosophical movements in Europe, the Reformation and the Enlightenment. The former is associated with individual conscience, individual responsibility, and the work ethic. The latter is associated with
confidence in reason and knowledge in human affairs. Thus, it was easy
to cope with the assertion that the current display of corruption and folly
was the result of decay. Original man, as created by God, uncorrupted
by evil, ignorant of both sin and folly, innocent in nakedness, might
yet exist and even, perhaps, have been discovered in the New World.

It was no accident of literary fantasy that Voltaire's Candide found
his way to a land of perfect innocence and extreme wealth and that the
land was El Dorado, literally "The Golden."

Rousseau and other writers of his time found proof of the perfection
of "primitive" man—and thereby the cause of their contemporaries
imperfections—in the governance of the indigenous peoples of the Eastern Seaboard of North America. The Europeans were convinced that
the scene of the perfect social contract had, in fact, been discovered.
They were made aware, largely through the work of Ben Franklin at
the Court of Louis XVI, of the structure of the League of the Iroquois.
Since Ben had a large hand in framing the tripartite form of government
created in 1789 in our own United States, there are serious scholars who
believe that the idea for the balance of power concept in our own govern-
mental structure came not from pure philosophy alone, but from admira-
tion and respect for the Iroquois Confederacy.

All this discussion of history emphasizes that the young people of the
communes are not the first to find an enviable life-style in the American
Indian societies of yesterday and today. Nor are they the only ones to
develop this interest. Others besides the young people have made books

about Indian culture (especially if accompanied by a small but intense dose of mysticism) the hottest selling items in the American book publishers' list.

We are all on a big Indian kick, and I, for one, am glad of it. Our technology has largely and inevitably replaced theirs. But the intangible elements of their belief systems and the web of interpersonal relationships continue functioning in the face of pressures that, in theory, ought to have demolished them a century ago.

The viability of these intangibles has caught the imagination of the younger generation, who see in it a chance to do what you and I have not done: to make a world you and I have not made and to do it with a minimum of help from you and me. We ignore and put down this hope at our peril.

These young people or their older siblings, sat down at a lunch counter in South Carolina some 15 years ago and started the Civil Rights revolt. They turned their attention to the war in Southeast Asia, forced a President out of office, and eventually forced withdrawal from Vietnam. The campuses are quiet, but the communes go on . . . and somebody is buying all those books about American Indian life. Who, I wonder? We, or they?

Communication and
the Deaf Patient

Luther D. Robinson, M.D., Sc.D.

Communication is among the most important activities of human beings. It is essential for personality development of the individual as well as for interpersonal relationships. For communication in our society we depend primarily on verbal language, both vocal and written. Even for the functionally illiterate, verbal-vocal language makes day-to-day communication possible. It is safe to say, therefore, that for the hearing society, communication is mainly an audio-vocal procedure, and, therefore, is based largely on an individual's ability to hear and speak. This rule holds true even internationally. However, if we are to perfect communication we must seek to understand one's culture as well as his language and, of course, there must be mutual understanding. Short of this understanding there must be mutual understanding of the commonalities among people of different nationalities, cultures, and subcultures. I became vividly aware of this about 23 years ago when as a military psychiatrist I was stationed in Japan during the Korean Conflict. For approximately 12 months, I was in charge of a 32-bed closed ward of psychiatric casualties from the armed forces of approximately eight different United Nation member countries. It was amazing to experience the order that existed in this situation, which could otherwise have been a Tower of Babel. Over many years I have had a chance to reflect on the commonalities that made such living successful. Among them were (1) the survival need, (2) the need or desire for gregariousness, (3) the need to be treated with human kindness (pleasure), and (4) to be recognized and treated with dignity as human beings.

Considering communication further one needs to view the role that communication plays in the development of the personality of the child. Even before the hearing infant can perceive language, he gets certain cues from his mother that give him a feeling of love, security, and comfort. These feelings are communicated through holding, caressing, feeding, and other aspects of mothering. There is even the bonus with sound, which the child can perceive in the mother's friendly, tender voice or in her footsteps approaching. Of course certain sounds can be frightening, and the infant learns to cope with them and distinguish them from friendly sounds. These factors all tend to facilitate the development of the child's personality.

With the deaf child, however, even though he may get the feeling of comfort through the caressing, feeding, and other aspects of mothering, he misses the added communications perceived by the hearing infant through the sound mechanism. This situation, of course, means that this one aspect of communication does not go into the development of the deaf child's personality. Moreover, with the deaf infant it is more than likely that the handicap will affect the parent/child relationship in the mothering of that child unless, however, the parent is a very unusual one. It would then appear that the deaf child would have much more to cope with in developing a normal personality than would the hearing child. It is as if the deaf child has two strikes against him at the start. This disadvantage is further aggravated by a not too uncommon procedure of removing the deaf child from the family at an early age and placing him in an institution for the deaf. To be sure, this kind of separation in itself would not facilitate communication between parents and child besides the other problematic effects it may have on the future attitudes and behavior of the child.

Since deaf people live in a hearing world, it is necessary to prepare them to compete with their hearing peers for all of the benefits to which they are entitled in a hearing society. One way to prepare the deaf individual is through education. Though educating the deaf child is one of the great accomplishments, there is still a great deal of controversy as to procedures and techniques to use in education. A perennial issue is the oral versus the manual method of communicating, and neither one at best is complete as compared with vocal language. It is generally agreed that the major percentage of our learning comes through hearing. It is, therefore, understandable that the deaf child may be at least two years behind his hearing peers as far as education is concerned, but beyond this it is also understandable that he may be behind his hearing peers in social aspects of living. This disadvantage is even compounded by the manner in which our industrial society regards the deaf individual and stereotypes and underemploys him in the work-a-day world of business and professions. Deafness is indeed a handicapped condition, but it does not exempt the individual from the same physical and mental problems of hearing people. Indeed the deaf person finds much more difficulty getting help for his physical and mental problems than does the hearing person because of the communication barrier. This difficulty does not necessarily mean that deaf people have more mental health problems than hearing people simply because of deafness. However, when they do have mental health problems these problems may be more difficult to detect or treat. Hearing people who are trained to treat mental illness are not usually trained in the particular technique of communicating with deaf people and therefore have difficulty bringing about a proper therapeutic relationship with deaf patients.

It is well to understand that the method deaf people use in communication depends largely upon the kind and extent of their education and training in language skills and concepts. Contrary to popular belief, all deaf people do not communicate by the language of signs. In fact, as mentioned, there are two opposing schools of thought on the methods of communication to be used by deaf people, viz., the oral versus the manual method. The oral method makes use of lip or speech reading by detecting words from the shapes made by a speaker's lips. Sign language is not a word-by-word substitute for verbal language but it has a conceptual quality. Low verbal deaf people use sign language and pantomime more so than high verbal deaf people who use more finger spelling. Also contrary to popular belief, deaf people have achieved higher academic degrees and more and more are earning degrees at the doctorate level. Reading and writing are also widely used by deaf people. Even in the writings of low verbal deaf, the sentence structure is so disordered that it is difficult to understand. Thus we can see that communication with deaf people through language can be a combination of techniques and the best combination should be used. We must also be aware that communication is more than verbal language exchange. Thus, there must be a mutual understanding between deaf patient and hearing therapist to facilitate communication.

Before going further, it is well to explain what we mean by deafness in terms of the people so affected. Realizing that it is not prudent to stereotype any group of people, it is safe to say that for the purposes of this paper, deaf people are those people whose hearing is so severely impaired that they depend primarily on other than auditory means for communication. Beyond this, for sake of clarity, we must separate the adventitiously deaf from the congenitally deaf and those who lost their hearing before they acquired vocal language. This paper addresses itself primarily to the latter two groups who pose the greater problem in terms of needs. Members of these groups frequently have the same life style, such as growing up in institutions for the deaf or attending other special schools or classes for the deaf and living a clannish type of life in a so-called "deaf community." Of course, few, if any, conditions exist in pure culture. Accordingly, all deaf people do not identify themselves with the deaf community but even some post-lingually deaf people do so identify themselves. In addition, just as in any group, wide individual variations exist with regard to language and intellectual ability and socio-economic status.

We have reason to believe that the incidence of mental illness within the deaf population is of the same order of magnitude as among the hearing, which is 1 to 10. Therefore, with the deaf population being approximately 350,000, we would estimate that about 35,000 deaf people have mental health problems. Over the years and until recently, very little help was available for the deaf mentally ill except custodial care in a mental institution. However, among pioneering programs are those by Kallman, Rainer, and Altshuler in New York, Grinker, Vernon, and Mindel in Chicago, and Robinson in Washington, D.C. A few others have subsequently developed.

I shall describe the Program that started at Saint Elizabeth's Hospital in Washington, D.C., in 1963. The Program is a pioneering effort that integrates services, training, and research, and combines communication techniques to provide optimum treatment and care for deaf patients. From a single activity of group psychotherapy for a small group of deaf patients in different sections of the Hospital, it developed over a three-year period into a full range of mental health services. These services include inpatient, outpatient, partial hospitalization, emergency, and diagnostic services; also consultation, education and training, research and evaluation, precare, aftercare, and rehabilitative services. It draws upon many different disciplines providing services in areas of psychiatry, general medicine, psychology, social service, nursing, psychodrama, individual and group psychotherapy, family therapy and marriage counseling, recreational therapy, creative drama, art, dance therapy, lip reading and sign language training, education and educational rehabilitation, occupational therapy, industrial therapy, vocational rehabilitation, hearing rehabilitation and speech therapy, medication, volunteer services, home arts, and religious ministry. Other services are continually being developed.

The Mental Health Program for the Deaf at Saint Elizabeth's Hospital has developed and expanded over the past 10 years to the point that now there is a patient load of approximately 81 patients. Of these patients, 35 were living in the hospital as of February, 1974, and the remaining 46 were living outside with family members or in a halfway house. The staff consists of 36 full-time members including a psychiatrist, clinical psychologist, social worker, educational therapist, rehabilitation personnel, clerical personnel, and nursing personnel. In addition, other hospital staff members devote full or part time to the Program.

The Program also serves as a training base for deaf and hearing people. On-the-job training in sign language and finger spelling and psychosocial aspects of deafness are provided for all workers on the Program. In addition, training, accredited by appropriate training schools and programs in various fields, is provided to satisfy their curriculum requirements. Research in this developing field has been in the area of (1) developing adequate psychological procedures for testing deaf people, (2) making demographic studies of deafness, and (3) developing the process of doing sleep studies in deafness.

In summary:

(a) Deaf people experience mental health problems similar to those of hearing people, but the communication difficulties make these mental health problems difficult to detect and treat.

(b) Few mental health services are available to deaf people throughout the country.

(c) In recent years some attention has been given to this problem, and services are gradually developing.

(d) Saint Elizabeth's Hospital has over the past 10 years carried out a mental health program that integrates services, training, and research and combines communication techniques to provide optimum treatment and care for the deaf.

(e) The author is of the opinion that many deaf patients and their families have benefited from this program and hopes that more programs of this nature will develop throughout the country to meet the mental health needs of deaf people.

(f) Although the Saint Elizabeth's Hospital Mental Health Program for the Deaf started independently, it recognizes a state of interdependence with the community, organizations, and agencies serving the deaf as it strives to achieve maximum benefit in the interest of improving the mental health of deaf people. Success of these very important efforts promises to lead to new insights in the field of mental health and of deafness.

Effective Communication in Adolescent Group Psychotherapy

Fern J. Azima, Ph.D.

Effective communication in the context of this presentation is meant to be the intellectual and emotional dialogues, verbal and nonverbal, amongst peers and therapists that are reciprocally understood and accepted, and that lead to better coping behavior on the part of the disturbed adolescent. Much "talk," explanation, and interpretation that may appear particularly wise from the therapist's point of view may be ineffective if it does not correspond to the needs of young members in the group, i.e., if the communication does not penetrate and touch the core of the problem. In the long run, one judges the effectiveness of the therapy communication by the attendance, or lack of it, and the gradual building of group cohesion and loyalty and changes in the group members that enable generalizing to the home, school, friends, and community.

The process of a well-functioning group leads to the gradual building of trust and intimacy that permit the risk of self-disclosure, critical self-examination, and the search for new solutions to reoccurring problems.

There appear to be certain general requirements for effective group leadership as well as other specific communication difficulties that are encountered by therapists who work with adolescents. A useful strategy for therapists working with adolescents would be: (1) to define a general model of the group leader's responsibilities, and (2) to catalog some of the specific impediments for both adolescent peers and the therapist that prevent effective communication. The goal, then, is to identify the specific impediments and distorted transference relationships and to strive to alter and modify them sufficiently so that each member can participate in an open dialogue and maintain greater pleasure and self-esteem. From the methodological point of view the therapist combines the interaction pattern of each member, the styles of initiation and reciprocation in the social matrix hierarchy, and the modification of the specific communication distortions for each member.

A General Model of Group Leadership

For some time there has been a heated controversy as to the qualifications of an effective group therapist. Some have stressed the cognitive factors: interpretation and working through; others the emotional warmth and empathy (Truax and Carkhuff, 1967) of the leader as being the major curative factors. It is the therapist's actual interactive mode in the group that mirrors how he thinks or feels, how he deals with distorted information, and how he encourages members to feel less negatively and to problem-solve more accurately. Unlike conventional leaders he makes no bid for power, his status does not have to be maintained by overbinding group members to him. He searches out the silent and negative members with the understanding that they cannot "repay" his initiations. At the same time, he must be concerned with the group as an effective ongoing, growing unit and makes timed references to the group as a whole. Much evidence exists to support that the therapist is a major builder of friendliness and group cohesion, while never forgetting his job of undoing faulty distortions and defenses and to allow the group to experiment in the present reality with new coping patterns that bring praise and growth in self-esteem. As the peers modify roles and status in the group, they assume greater influence, responsibility, and independence in working through their own problems.

Specific Communication Difficulties in Adolescent Groups

In a strict context the problems of peer transference and leader countertransference are the essence of the marked difficulties that hinder and block ineffective communication. Transference as such may be described as the repetitive, unconscious, emotionally significant manifestations of patient behavior in relation to the therapist, to other group members, and to the group as a whole. "From this point of view transference stretches horizontally in the present and vertically in time, and integrates both intrapsychic and interpersonal phenomena. The multiplicity of interrelationships in the group structure identifies a different monitoring system, and alters significantly the reflective attitudes of reciprocating patient and leader'' (Azima, 1973). Countertransference may be defined as the therapist's repetitive, unconscious-motivated, conflictual response to the individual patient or to the pressures of the group as a whole. The therapist who has an overabundance of such irrational communications cannot deal objectively or effectively with the group. At the same time it is inconceivable that some manifestations of countertransference reactions are not alerted by the adolescent culture. With this proviso, the following examples are termed as transference, inasmuch as they stem from past, unconscious, distorted reactions that are repeated and reactivated in the here-and-now, and continue to hinder the socialization process.

Transference Themes in Adolescent Groups. This discussion will briefly review: attitudes towards authority and peers, acting out, silence, and somatization.

Attitudes Towards Authority and Peers. In an early group session the following dialogue took place:

MEMBER 1: Why should I go to school? The courses are lousy, they don't interest me, and the teachers are always on my back.

MEMBER 2: I agree, they sit so smugly, worrying only about their paycheques and not us.

THERAPIST: And here—you expect the same?

MEMBER 1: Well, you should know better.

MEMBER 3: But I do like the fact that here I can listen to the opinions of kids my own age—and the group is exclusively for us, and my parents can't butt in.

THERAPIST: You are all probably fearful and distrusting for good reason, and worried whether your parents will control you as in the past. I can't promise that everything will be perfect here, but remember it is not your home or school here and we have a chance to size up if we are seeing things clearly.

The therapist's response above was an attempt to prevent an identification with the nagging parent and to orient them to the here-and-now and to set the goal of reclarification. It is of some interest to note Member 1's change over the last 5 months. This 16-year-old, intelligent, passive-rebelling girl had been out of school for the past 6 months. In a recent session she said:

MEMBER 1: I really am surprised how much better it is at school and how well my work is going. Even that bloody principal smiles at me differently.

MEMBER 2: Fantastic, and how about at home?

MEMBER 1: Even with my father it is 100% better. When I say how was work today, he really knows I meant it and really talks "to me." I'd like to tell you that my kid brother who has the learning difficulties came home the other day after a gym day with a lot of ribbons. I was glad for the ribbons, but I really was happy for him. For the first time I could feel something else except rage and jealousy.

THERAPIST: Even as you talk now we all can see your spontaneity and your pride. It is a lot different than when you were so distrustful, angry, and moody.

MEMBER 3: I wish I could relate to my family the same way. I just hate them.

The above vignettes demonstrate how one member has lifted some of the blocks in communication in the group, in her home, and at school. She has become a highly influential member encouraging others to risk "opening up" and setting new goals. The therapist must accept anger and criticism without becoming irrational and overemotional as have authority figures in the past. However, it is very important to recognize that the therapist must not join in the open rage against the parent. If the therapist condemns the parent, the adolescent will retaliate by breaking treatment. One admits that many authority figures have marked difficulties of their own, but they are not in the present treatment group and the goal is for modification in their own behavior to improve communication with others on more independent, less distorted levels. The improving adolescents become (as Member 1 above) cotherapists.

An example from a session in the fourth month is illustrative of libidinal peer transference behavior. Bruce was a tall, blond, sulking, self-centered boy who always sat with his jacket on. He rarely listened to others, always believed he was right and the authority in all areas. It was clear there was some ambivalence between Bruce and Claire, a most attractive, dark-haired girl who sighed every time he began his boastful exposés.

BRUCE: You are just the kind of rich snob I can't stand. So much makeup, and look at your clothes and your jewelry. Those rings and watch. I can just see you brushing every guy off like dust.

CLAIRE: You are stupid—Rich—ha—my mother is a maid and I've got nothing to be stuck up about. I'm even an illegitimate child.

The group members pointed out that he was really attracted to Claire, but that he was afraid she would not give him a tumble. The therapist at this early stage did not interpret this adolescent's constant fear of rejection (his mother would not keep him) and his fragile sexual identity. (He had been picked up by the police for homosexual loitering.) It was clear to the group that this attack was distorted and revealing of his past unresolved problems.

Acting Out. Adolescents are known for their normal capricious acting out and this in itself alerts many rigid therapists to become very defensive in dealing with teenagers. What is of more importance from the psychotherapeutic point of view is to identify the transferential compulsive acting out and repetitive defense based upon a variety of historical unsatisfied needs.

Nancy, an 18-year-old, talked openly in the group of her sexual acting out, chronic use of hard and soft drugs, and her numerous suicidal attempts. She was an intelligent, powerful group member who was highly skilled in identifying and interpreting the behavior of other group members. In several sessions she threatened to leave the city. At the same time she had taken to telephoning various members in the group. In one specific session the following conversation took place.

NANCY: Yes, really I am going to leave. I can't keep up the apartment, and my parents are throwing a fit about my relationship with Dick.

BOB: I think you are copping out again. You've tried every hospital, doctor, and social worker. You really are an important member to the group. You always help others but not yourself, and you are not giving us a chance to help you.

GROUP: (Many agreeing statements.)

CLAIRE: My mother got another phone call and she said it was somebody from the group.

NANCY: No, it wasn't me this time—honest. I have phoned you before.

MARY: But you did phone me.

SID: And me.

THERAPIST: Nancy, you seem to be kind of playing therapist outside of the group, and getting many people on your side. Do you think (addressed to the group) that she could be recruiting members to join her if she leaves the group?

There began an active discussion in which Nancy admitted her constant fear of getting involved anywhere for the repeated danger of being abandoned. She resisted with defiant determination that she could be helped. In fact this patient left the group for a month, but returned downcast, admitting guilt that one of the boys in the group had visited her but she had resisted. She was a high-risk patient whose self-destructive acting out was a constant danger for the group and encouraged dependency and overprotection. At the same time she must be confronted with her anger. As Mary told her recently: "You are just plain dumb and how long can you act this way?" The therapist commented that Mary was so angry because Nancy had helped so much in the past and was not letting her reciprocate.

Sometimes a powerful group member exploits a weaker one to act out her defiance, as for example when a girl threw the darts at the therapist at the provocation of another (see Azima, 1973). In this instance group pressure "saved" the therapist and helped expose the real culprit.

Body language and nonverbal behavior communicate a wide variety of acting out, e.g., head slapping, lighting matches, and actually burning fingers and clothing, scratching the furniture, etc.

Cultural patterns have changed considerably in the last twenty years. Previously many adolescents were excessively shy, inhibited, and guilt ridden. Schizoid adolescents still behave in this fashion, but most feel justified to act, disagree, fight the establishment and no longer to sulk in silent rage. Encounter techniques are not needed for this group; in fact, the need for control over primitive drives is often requested by the adolescents themselves.

Silence. Adolescents in the group poorly tolerate silence, even though they are the most excellent utilizers of this technique with parents and teachers. "Keep cool—give them the stony eye—not a word—not a flicker of interest." This routine is highly successful in raising the anger of the authority, and the therapist must not fall into this trap.

Silence is a resistance that clothes a variety of transferential fears, e.g., "I was afraid if I talked about what I did I would be the sickest person here'' (the patient walked in cemeteries in the dark of night collecting all the stray cats). For several months this obese girl sat with her coat wrapped around her. On the day she took her coat off the therapist asked if she was ready to ''open up,'' and she smiled and said yes. (Five years later she is a highly competent nurse.)

Another boy broke his silence after several months in a heated discussion of drugs. The therapist stated: ''No one gives up drugs if they really are greater than any other experience you can have.'' Stan attacked the therapist, saying that she should ''warn them of the consequences.'' The group, quickly alerted, asked Stan how he was so knowledgeable — and Stan answered: ''I'm a narc [narcotics agent] planted by the police in my school — and I've been afraid to tell you.'' The group was silent and then asked if he was informing on them. Stan quickly said, ''Of course not. I hate the job, but it's the only way I can deal with my father.'' It soon became clear that he became a more super detective than his military father. It was one way to have power over him and to disguise his own rebelliousness.

Many silent members talk with their eyes, a glare, raised eyebrows, mumbling, wincing, pursed lips, raised shoulders, tapping fingers or toes. To the latter behavior a therapist once caught a silent member off-guard by asking, ''What did you say? I didn't understand your morse code.'' To which the member responded, ''You're right, I do have something to say.''

A trap set by silent members is that other talkative peers and therapist do the talking for them. In this way the silent member never has to be responsible for the decisions made for him. Some therapists maintain that silent members do really get something from the group. A few may profit, for unless the patient regains the use of language and participates, there is no evidence of change. The transferential reasons for silence range from the defiant, sulking child, sadness, defiance, anger, fear of loss of control, fear of giving, etc. Many times a silent member wields significant power in the group and frequently is encouraged covertly by peers not to talk but to act out a group resistance whether it be sadness, rage, fear, etc. He is asked to be the hold-out for their own defensive fears.

Somatization. The technique of handling stress by individual members is usually seen by the somatic symptoms actually noticed or discussed in the group. Fainting, hyperventilation, headache, sweating, asthma attacks, palpitations, seizures, encopresis and vomiting are but a few seen by the author. Often both patient and therapist cling tenaciously to the discussion of the symptoms as a defense to prevent coming to grips with emotional problems. In my own experience adolescents are not so preoccupied with somatic symptoms to the degree of adult patients, and their wish is for health, not illness.

The therapist's technique may be seen from the following example of nail-biting. Ann sat biting her nails as Bob watched her.

BOB:	You bite them?
ANN:	Yes, I like to.
SANDRA:	You suck them?
ANN:	No, I eat my nails.
THERAPIST:	You don't chew them down very far. They don't even bleed.
ANN:	No, I don't like to hurt myself.
SANDRA:	Have you tried to stop?
ANN:	I can't.

In this example the therapist demonstrates that she allies early in therapy with the impulse, is not perturbed, and allows the patients to verbalize without fear of parental chastisement. The peers soon discover that there is no active witch hunt against symptoms, which disappear as tension, anger, and loneliness decrease.

At times hyperventilation, asthma attacks, running to the toilet, and feeling sick occur in the group when relevant transferential figures are discussed or "taboo" topics that the members have not been able to reveal. A common feature of all transference reactions is the defensive nature of continuing to raise patterns of behavior to prevent self-disclosure of their bad and sinful thoughts and feelings. Once these are exposed and the patient is not ostracized or rejected, and feared catastrophe does not result, they experience relief from symptoms, gratification, and acceptance.

Countertransference Reactions of Therapists. Countertransference reactions in therapists are often quickly mobilized by adolescents who invade their privacy, show lack of respect, attack, and "fool around." Beginning therapists often complain that adolescents are not serious enough, and miss that the essence of adolescent communication is contained in this playful, acting out, defiant behavior. Therapists unwilling or unable to be in touch with their own adolescent feelings do not enjoy the expressing of their own spontaneity, and become overserious, rejecting, and intolerant of regressive behavior of the patients. "The dilemma clearly posed for the therapist working with adolescents is how to maintain an intermediate position in the chronological and maturational ladders; he will never be accepted as a peer, and he should not retreat into an autocratic judgemental role" (Azima, 1973).

Some therapists are further ineffective communicating with adolescents in that they have low frustration tolerance for anger, acting out for fear that it will unmask their own adolescent rebelliousness. They stifle the group and overdemand conformity. The over-scientific status approach is often a way to mask fears of shame, inferiority, and helplessness.

Many therapists are helped in supervision in overcoming their unrecognized countertransference reactions. The interrelated issues of omnipotence, fear of self-disclosure, overidentification with the adolescent, somatizations, and blind spots will be very briefly reviewed.

Omnipotence. Omnipotent therapists encourage dependency and prevent autonomous growth. The therapist who needs to be too brilliant and too powerful prevents the patient from seeking solutions for himself and quite frequently causes withholding, e.g., "Since you know everything even before I say it, why bother?". The therapist is afraid to look weak and vulnerable. He is unable to admit he can make mistakes. His over-perfectionism blocks competition since the adolescent soon senses that if they "argue" or disagree, the therapist's narcissism will be hurt. At the same time, the omnipotent overambitious therapist insists on the "best group," the fastest cures, and cannot tolerate failure easily.

It is important to note that the adolescents in the early stages of treatment push for an omnipotent all-saving therapist. Therapists who cannot admit their limitations will maintain dependent, helpless patients. The transferential dream of regaining the perfect parent or savior must be exposed. An omnipotent therapist may vary from being exhibitionistic and overly assertive on the one hand, to being overly silent, distant, and mysterious, maintaining the image of the silent sage and the only one in the group possessed with the capacity of understanding.

Fear of Self-disclosure. All group therapists have become more active in group interaction in the last decade. The dilemma is clearly that the more active the therapist becomes the more he self-discloses and tends to find himself vulnerable. The professional, distant calm of the overneutral therapist is a way to keep in check exposure of his own aggressive and libidinal drives. The therapist who must overprotect the public image of himself is usually too rigid and fearful, and raises the anger of the adolescent.

A well-known defense overused by therapists in the past is to answer a question with a question, especially if it is one that encroaches on his own privacy. Adolescents are highly skillful in such invasion tactics. The calm, flexible therapist answers many questions about himself and draws a line at the point where he wants to further encroachment. The fifth-amendment rule is a good safeguard for both therapist and peers to protect their personal selves under the attack of group pressure.

Overidentification with the adolescent. At the other extreme some therapists develop an overcloseness and intimacy with the adolescents, behaving almost as peers. At first adolescents also like the "good guy" approach, but soon they will become alarmed by the overcloseness and the often implied seductiveness, voyeurism, and become aware of the therapists' vicarious need to relive their own adolescence. Starting with overidentification, therapists have difficulty in setting an adult model to which the adolescent should maturate. Adolescents quickly manipulate the overly permissive hippie therapist who can set no rules.

Sometimes, it is quite difficult to see that some quiet, conservative therapists are involved in such overidentification with the adolescents. The following example may be illustrative. Two analytically oriented therapists started a group in a home for delinquent boys. They were quiet, neutral, attentive, and showed little emotional response to the anger of the boys. Their leaders did state that "some of the rules and regulations here are difficult." In the third session the boys destroyed the entire group room. In supervision it became clear that the therapists had given the message that they were on the boys' side and against the "establishment." Since they set no rules or gave no emotional response themselves, they gave tacit assent for the boys to escalate their anger and to act out viciously their own desires to get rid of the bad place.

There is no such thing as completely neutral behavior. Every therapist communicates even by his "hmms," shrugs, body geography, and eyes whether he is in agreement or disagreement, and if he wishes the conversation to continue. Sexual countertransference may underlie some of the therapist's difficulties and are disguised by his coldness, vagueness, or openly evidenced by his overconcern. The therapist must be secure enough in his own sexual role not to become overly provocative or seductive, or at the other extreme a cold fish. Spontaneity and a good sense of humor are important parts of the therapist's emotional repertoire with adolescents.

Somatizations and Blind Spots. The therapist becomes alerted to his own anxiety or depression by symptoms such as headaches, flushing, nausea, cramps, urinary frequency, etc. Yawning and falling asleep may be due at times to fatigue but most often when analyzed are related to flight from anger and attack.

Therapists only become aware of their blind spots by being observed from behind a one-way screen or in group supervision when peers identify behavior that has not been otherwise reported. A supervisor who listens only to retrospective reports or audiotapes is often significantly surprised when he watches his supervisee on video or in reality.

In conclusion, the paper has had the goal of presenting a general model of the effective group therapist and his major responsibilities for both cognitive and positive emotional leadership. In addition, some specific transference reactions for adolescents and countertransference reactions of the therapist were outlined, which impair communication. It is felt that this cataloging may be helpful to the therapist who wishes to promote effective communication in adolescent groups. In addition, however, to adequate skills and experience and a minimum of countertransference reactions, certain personality characteristics in the group therapist appear essential and those include spontaneity, enthusiasm, optimism, trust, honesty, a sense of humor, and affection for and belief in the integrity of the young.

REFERENCES

Azima, Fern J. (1974). Behavioral Indices of Individual and Group Dynamics. *International Journal of Group Psychotherapy.*

Azima, Fern J. (1973). *Transference —Countertransference in Group Therapy for the Adolescent.* eds. N. S. Brandes and M. L. Gardner. New York: Jason Aronson, Inc. pp. 101–26.

Azima, Fern J. (1972). Transference-Countertransference Issues in Group Psychotherapy for Adolescents. *International Journal of Child Psychology,* 1, 4, 51–70.

Bales, R. F. (1950). *Interaction Process Analysis: A Method for the Study of Small Groups*. Cambridge, Mass.: Addison-Wesley.

Psathas, G. (1960). Interaction Process Analysis of Two Psychotherapy Groups. *This Journal,* 10, 430–45.

Talland, G. A. (1955). Task and Interaction Process: Some Characteristics of Therapeutic Group Discussion. *Journal of Abnormal and Social Psychology,* 50, 105–09.

Truax, C. and Carkhuff, E. (1967). *Toward Effective Counselling and Psychotherapy*. New York: Aldine Publishing Co.

The Machine as Diagnostician and Therapist

Lewey O. Gilstrap, Jr.

Introduction

The complex processes of diagnosis and therapy can be aided by the use of machines. Medical science, in fact, abounds with a great variety of machines, instruments, and implements. (For the sake of having a generic term, we will refer to instruments and implements as machines.) Based on experience and knowledge, a physician selects among these available machines those most appropriate for some immediate problem at hand.

From a historical view, the number of machines available to the physician is increasing. Even the rate of increase is increasing, and, looking to the future, one is prompted to ask how long this trend will go on and what the situation might be like some years from now. For example, will the time come when more and more of the task of diagnosis is or could be turned over to machines? This paper is concerned with recent developments in theoretical and mathematical techniques that can be used for diagnosis.

Therapy is also often machine aided for a variety of conditions. The primary concern with therapy in this paper is the use of physiological monitoring devices whose outputs are fed back to patients for self-corrective action; in short, biofeedback. In particular, the information-theoretic basis for biofeedback, which is seldom discussed, will be described.

Diagnosis

There is an axiom in the field of automation to the effect that if a process is to be automated, it must first be completely systematized and regularized: every step in the process must be precisely and unambiguously defined. This axiom does not imply that an automated process is a rigid or inflexible one, with no variation allowed with changing conditions. If there are variations in the process, the tests required to make the decision as to how to modify the process and the alternatives in processing must be defined.

Systematizing a process need not automatically imply that a machine, such as a computer, is required to carry out the process. The decision to convert a systematized manual process into a machine process is (or should be) based on unit cost of manual and machine output and on total volume of output desired or required, assuming that other factors, such as quality of the output, are not appreciably different for manual and machine processing. In principle, the *last* thing to be decided in automating is the choice of a computer or machine to do the work; a machine might be unnecessary and unwarranted.

Some processes are so complex that no one has ever succeeded in completely systematizing them. However, the processes are understood and they can be taught. The above is simply a reflection of the gap that exists between human comprehension or ability to do things and the human ability to explain why they do certain things. The gifted artist, the master craftsman, the composer, the chess grand master, and the diagnostician are all examples of human beings who have mastered a process they can use but who have not been perfectly replicated by a machine.

The development of practical machines that can acquire information about an imperfectly defined process and can use this information to improve the machine performance (in short, machines that learn or learning machines) which has taken place in the last ten or fifteen years has changed the situation markedly, however. These machines, or rather specialized computer software and hardware, have already been used to match or exceed human performance in some control processes that have previously resisted automation. Machines that learn have great promise of handling the problem of diagnosis. Technically, it now appears feasible to develop a comprehensive diagnostic program for computerization. Whether it is desirable to do so is another matter. Even a computer program that learns to diagnose more accurately than its human teachers might be objected to on the grounds that it is "inhuman" or "unfeeling."

It must be stated that the process of diagnosis is quite complex, and although there have been experimental computer programs for diagnosis, none have thus far approached being satisfactory. In this paper the key mathematical elements needed in a diagnosis program will be described.

Every diagnosis starts with the acquisition of information, from interrogation, direct examination, and tests. In principle, all information can be reduced to binary form suitable for entry into a computer by expressing the information as a set of "yes-no" answers to questions. Measures and numerical values can be entered directly into a computer, so that both qualitative and quantitative information can be fed to the computer. The question is what the computer can do with such information, once it is entered, since the computer cannot think or reason.

The simplest thing the computer can do is to provide to a diagnostician ready access to statistical information: out of some total number of cases with roughly similar characteristics, a certain percentage had one condition, while another percentage had a different condition, and so on. While diagnosticians generally already have statistical information of this type as part of their general knowledge and make use of it in arriving at a diagnosis, it is not decisive information, and the clinician has a number of options to resolve uncertainty, such as ordering further tests or keeping the patient under observation to allow the condition to develop to a later stage where it may be more easily identified. In any event, a statistical summary is only a collection of odds, it is not a decision-making system.

A mathematical decision function can be constructed from the same historical information used to construct statistical summaries. Since the same data can be used in either case, it might be concluded that a decision function could do no better than simply taking the highest probability condition. Such a conclusion would not be correct, however, because a decision function must take into account the risk of possible errors in making decisions. Also, it is now possible to construct highly nonlinear decision functions that can handle hundreds of measurements and observations. These nonlinear decision functions can often do a remarkably accurate job of separating two similar conditions, and they are essential if the computer is ever to be used in diagnosis as anything more than a records keeper.

Because the nonlinear functions are so effective in separating conditions with similar symptoms, some of the mathematical aspects of their construction will now be summarized. If the observational data and measurements taken from patients with similar conditions were to be plotted, it could be observed that the data would tend to form a cluster. If there are a total of n observations and measurements, the data would have to be plotted on n-dimensional graph paper, which cannot, of course, be realized or visualized, but can be accomplished with mathematical techniques. Some variables will be extraneous for a given condition, and there will be no tendency for the data to cluster along extraneous dimensions.

Data corresponding to a second condition will tend to form slightly different clusters. For either or both conditions, the clusters will generally tend to be irregular in shape, most probably with some overlap in the clusters if the two conditions are similar (as determined from the measurements and observations, not from the underlying anatomical or physiological conditions). As a general rule, the greater the number of observations or measurements of relevant variables, the better the separation between clusters.

The surface that separates two or more such clusters (technically, a *hypersurface* if more than three measurements are used) is called a *decision boundary* when it is used for separation of classes. Although a number of figures with simple geometrical shape have been used for decision boundaries, such as spheres, ellipsoids and planes, the most satisfactory for irregular-shaped clusters is simply a nonlinear hypersurface.

The practical construction of arbitrary, nonlinear hypersurfaces has been achieved only within the past ten years. Even though nonlinear hypersurfaces can be applied to a large number of extremely complex problems, such as diagnosis, the practical realization of these mathematical functions required the solution to some extraordinary problems. Because these problems are indicative of the power of the nonlinear hypersurface, they will be reviewed briefly.

Fitting hypersurface to arbitrary data is much like fitting a curve to data; in fact, it is the n-dimensional generalization of curve fitting, and the same basic problems must be solved in either case. The basic steps include selecting a criterion of goodness of fit, finding the values of a set of coefficients, and avoiding overfitting the data. There is a major difference between hypersurface approximation and curve fitting, however. If the nth degree algebraic polynomial is fitted to data, only $n+1$ constants must be determined, and these constants can be found by simple matrix inversion. The number of constants that must be computed for a hypersurface depends on the number of variables (total number of measurements and observations) and on the degree of the highest degree term: the number, N_c, of constants is equal to $\dfrac{(n + d)!}{n!d!}$, where n is the number of variables and d is the degree of the highest degree term. This factorial expression increases at a great rate. For example, if the number of variables is one and the highest degree term is the fifth power, only 6 constants must be found; this is the case of curve fitting. If 5 variables are involved, and the highest degree term is fifth, then 252 constants must be found. If 24 variables to fifth degree are to be found, the number of coefficients is 118,755. This last example is not just an academic illustration. The first practical problem solved by hypersurface approximation had 24 variables to the fifth degree.

There is a general rule in algebra to the effect that if there are N variables to be solved for, at least N equations must be used. Yet only about 50 pieces of information were needed to solve that particular problem, and 25 were sufficient to do a fairly good job. This characteristic of needing only a small amount of data to fit a hypersurface with very high variability is extremely important for such problems as diagnosis, where there is a limited amount of data on some conditions and more than needed on others.

Without digressing into the mathematics of hyperspace, it is not possible to prove here that it is quite practical to fit hypersurfaces with a small amount of data, far less than expected from the general rules for solving simultaneous linear equations. (See Reference for a discussion of the mathematics.) By way of nonmathematical explanation, however, the reason why the method works is that the intrinsic variability in most complex natural problems is not nearly so great as the number of coefficients in a general multinomial (polynomial in many variables). The way the hypersurface approximation method works, the hypersurface may be highly nonlinear and require many constants. But these constants need not all be (and are not) independent, so that a small set of independent constants can be used to construct the very much larger number needed for a hypersurface.

The method of fitting hypersurfaces is now very much refined, and one very important feature has been incorporated. This feature is the avoidance of overfitting. Frequently, in using regression, one finds that a data base can be fitted very well, but the regression gives very poor results when used with new data. This phenomenon is quite real, and it has been given the name *overfitting*. Present methods of fitting hypersurfaces completely avoid overfitting, and a fitted hypersurface will give consistent results (within 1 to 2 percent) when applied to new data. Needless to say, overfitting of data in diagnosis can be highly misleading if not dangerous.

The method for avoiding overfitting makes use of an iterative, stochastic fitting procedure that, in action, resembles trial-and-error learning. The terms ''learning machine'' and ''computer programs that learn'' are derived from the similarity of the stochastic process to learning.

At this time, hypersurface approximation has been used on a very wide variety of problems and, although no two data bases are alike, some general conclusions can be given about this technique. First, its accuracy equals or exceeds that of a skilled human being making decisions based on training and experience. Second, it generally takes less information in a data base for the computer to build up an acceptable decision function than it does for the human being. It must be added that the time required to make a decision using a hypersurface decision boundary requires only a fraction of a second on a small computer, once the measurements have been loaded.

Despite the advance in machine capability for diagnosis represented by hypersurface approximation, this technique still falls short of what a human being can do. The nonlinear decision function can only be obtained from historical data, and the computer can reach no conclusion as to diagnosis, treatment, or prognosis if it has never seen a given condition (except the bare conclusion that the case is unfamiliar, which is not altogether trivial). The human being also has a mental model of human structure and function and can often cope readily with conditions never before observed, simply by reasoning. The construction of a model of a human being of sufficient complexity and accuracy to be of assistance in machine diagnosis is quite probably feasible, although most certainly a task that could not be completed in any short period of time. It is possible that a machine learning feature would be of some value in reducing the amount of time required to construct such a model.

Returning to one of the questions raised in the introduction to this paper, i.e., when we might expect a diagnostic program aid, it is possible to speculate about the technical aspect of computerization. A program for diagnosis based on hypersurface approximation is only as good as the data used to develop the program. Constructing a good data base, reasonably complete and as free of errors as possible, is the most difficult part of the task. Given a large medical center with existing computerization of patient records, however, it should be possible in six months to a year to have an experimental diagnosis program turning out quite respectable diagnoses for a wide variety of ailments.

Computer programs for diagnosis have been written before, but none of these programs made use of hypersurface approximation. While it is difficult to estimate how accurate a diagnosis program based on hypersurface approximation will be as compared to a good human diagnostician, we can be quite certain that the program will be at least as good as the best program constructed using any other approach and will most likely be a great deal better.

Therapy

Research in the field of biofeedback is, for the most part, sober and cautious. While popularizations of this research tend to the sensational side, it nevertheless appears that biofeedback is already a useful therapeutic alternative that will become more valuable in the future. Biofeedback is the name popularly applied to the process of monitoring one or more physiological variables of a subject, such as scalp potentials, muscle potentials (including both heart potentials and skeletal muscle potentials), galvanic skin resistance, local temperatures in the body, and gastric acidity, and then displaying either the values of the variables or some thresholded measure of the variables to the subject, along with instructions as to how to modify the variables. The subject then learns how to produce the desired changes in the monitored variables, generally returning the values to a range more consistent with good health.

Generally, although not always, most subjects can learn some degree of conscious control over any or all of the above-listed variables. There is an apparent paradox here in that most of these variables are controlled by signals that must travel through the autonomic nervous system. Prior to the studies of conditioning of autonomic functions in the mid to late 1960s, it was generally assumed that conscious control of autonomically controlled processes in the body was not possible. Once it had been shown that curarized rats could be conditioned to vary heart rate and blood pressure on cue, the entire range of autonomic functions was suddenly fair game.

Empirical evidence aside, the big puzzle was how did it work, or even how could it possibly work. One thing became clear from biofeedback studies. The old identification of conscious control with striped muscles only and unconscious control with smooth muscles, glands, nerves, and almost everything else was no longer tenable. While it is not yet possible to give an account of consciousness or to answer the question of what can and cannot be consciously controlled, it is possible to give a partial account.

While the autonomic nervous system does not normally respond to conscious commands, it does respond to conscious evaluations of situations. The decision that a certain situation has just become dangerous, even without any overt signs, is apt to be followed by an increase in the output of adrenaline and other fright or flight reactions. Thus, it is clear that there are at least some pathways linking the conscious to the "unconscious" brain activities.

All of the more directly controllable striated muscles are addressable through the cerebellum. It would appear that the cerebellum organizes and coordinates striated muscle activity, and to oversimplify, that is its job. There is no corresponding organ to coordinate autonomic signals and to simplify their response to conscious control. Nevertheless, the control pathways do exist, even though a different sort of effort from that required to signal striped muscles is needed to produce action.

The autonomic system does, as it must, function automatically as a servo system, and the observation that the external situation can modify (but not control) the autonomic system implies only a linkage in set points, but not in direct control. While analogies can be misleading, we could, borrowing from the computer field, say that the cerebellum acts as an interpreter of a high-level language of the brain (e.g., the desire to pick up something or to walk to some point), whereas, there exists no high-level language interpreter for autonomic signals, and signals through the autonomic nervous system must be in a low level or machine language.

In any event, the brain and nervous system are fairly well self-connected; the nervous system qualifies as an anastomotic network of cells, meaning that information from any one part can travel to most other parts. This fact alone may be sufficient to account for conscious control of autonomic activity.

Whatever the final explanation for the feasibility of biofeedback training, empirically it speaks for itself. By now, it has been used as an adjunct in treating such varied functional disorders as simple headaches, migraine headaches, tics, muscle spasms, gastric hyperacidity, and to reduce the frequency of epileptic seizures, according to a variety of popular reports. However, research on therapeutic uses has barely begun. It is evident that the field will not fully develop until a fairly broad range of functions can be monitored simultaneously. At the discretion of the therapist, then appropriate signals could be fed back to the patient for adjustment. Combining the diagnostic power of hypersurface approximation with the self-corrective power of the human being, there appears to be little reason why a person might not some day be able to connect himself to a computer via appropriate sensors and get an automatic tune-up.

REFERENCES

Gilstrap, L. O., Jr. "Keys to Developing Machines with High-Level Artificial Intelligence." Presented to ASME Design Engineering Conference. New York, April 19–22, 1971 (ASME Paper #71-DE-21).

The Impact of the
Women's Liberation Movement
on Male Identity

Robert L. Vosburg, M.D.

Introduction

I was asked to present my impression of the effects of the Women's Liberation movement on male identity. The following address builds on a base of observations made of "normal" men between 30 and 50 years of age, married, and living in a variety of circumstances. The presentation here deals particularly with clinical observations drawn from interaction with my students, colleagues, and patients.

The Concept of Identity

Who am I? Who are you?

William James wrote to his wife (in the example selected by Erikson to illustrate *identity*):

A man's character is discernable in the mental or moral attitude in which, when it came upon him, he felt himself most deeply and intensely active and alive. At such moments there is a voice inside which speaks and says: "This is the real me!" The real me who is addressing you is a speaker, a clinician, a father, a lover, and a golfer. Yet to list such terms does not establish an identity. My identity derives from our interaction. Positive identity is in relationship to some countervailing force: viz: "The fearless freedom of thinking of the Jews contrasted with the negative trait in 'the peoples among whom we Jews live', namely, prejudices which restrict others in the use of intellect."[1]

Financially successful, white, middle-aged males have been the hero figures in our society. Through the 1960s student revolt and black activism challenged that tradition. Now women too revolt against the old hero, now termed a "male chauvinist pig." As a clinician I have observed many men who feel shattered by these assaults. I would like to be a spokesman today for their condition, especially to consider the basis for effective outpatient therapy.

The term "identity crisis" originated with Erik Erikson. It was used to describe patients returning from World War II "who had neither been shell shocked nor become malingerers, but had through the exigencies of war lost a sense of personal sameness and historical continuity." Erikson later extended the concept of loss of ego identity to apply to adolescents lost in confusion and rebellion, and still later to biographical reconstructions. In characteristic self-scrutiny Erikson freely admits he is unsure what identity "really is." Being the originator of the concept and committed to psychohistory, his answer to the public was a book, a compendium of his essays on identity written over a space of twenty years.[1] My own observations extend his views in a few particulars.

We may well ask if an opposing force to male identity is female liberation. If so, then it follows that male infants, boys, young men, mature adults, and aging fellows all must be threatened. My observations are limited to self-observation and those men whom I treat, the majority of whom are white, married, and between 20 and 50 years of age. About their lives I am familiar. We hear it said the middle-aged male faces a crisis of identity, but what that means is never clear. Recently I heard a man say that he felt like a bowl of cereal and that everyone has a spoon into him; that puts the matter graphically. Possibly young men and old men also feel consumed, but I shall leave their fate to other discussion.

The Concept of Crisis

One meaning of crisis is portrayed in the Chinese ideograph by combining two symbols, one standing for danger the other for opportunity. So a crisis is a time of danger and opportunity. Certainly men feel the danger, but rarely do they feel fresh opportunity. When a man blurts out he is a bowl of cereal, we understand his sense of self in relation to others. He implies he nourished others at the price of self extinction. To expand his metaphor of identity crisis I will present a case history and discuss some therapeutic opportunities. In these matters you may assume I practice what I preach.

This case history was presented by a woman about 24 years old who is a senior medical student A man about 35 years of age came to the walk-in-service in a panic. She described him as "looking like a movie star who's name I can't remember"; he looked strong, self-reliant. He spoke very rapidly and abstractly. Recently he had struck his wife and was appalled by what he had done. He went on to say his wife accuses him of being irresponsible. That means he won't help her out with household tasks. He complained he knew her accusation to be true but didn't know why. He wanted clarification for he felt overwhelmed and confused. Despite this panic reaction he was able to continue his work at the middle management level in a nearby business concern.

The history revealed that his wife had seemed very like his mother during the first several years of their 12-year marriage. Recently she has been different. He struck her during an argument about another man. Three years ago he had left another job in the city and had come to Vermont to run a ski resort. It was an attempt to please her and improve their marriage. His father years ago had done something rather similar. He had desired to be a chemist but went to medical school and then practiced medicine at the urging of the patient's mother. The practice had never been much of a success.

The student noted in the second interview this man's fear of hitting his wife seemed to represent a fear of losing control. His ramblings were countered by urging him to express his feelings and stick to the point. He said he has a problem of commitment: he feels uncommitted. Recently his wife wanted him to paint the house. He was afraid he'd make a mess of it. Actually the job turned out well. He was afraid of how it would look to the neighbors.

The student urged the wife to come to the third interview but she refused. She said, "I've had my say; you need to see the doctor!" The student urged him to renegotiate with his wife but the patient responded, "If I bargain I lose, because I must be strong in my work." One of the staff said at this point in the presentation, "What has he got that the wife wants anyway? That's the basis of bargaining!"

In the fourth interview the student focused upon decision making. When the patient said his wife had been self-effacing throughout the early years of the marriage, the student said, "That set you up to be criticized whenever anything went wrong." He felt much better as a result of that comment. In the fifth interview he commented that his wife sets up tasks for him and he lives by a rule that if he can't do the job perfectly, he won't do it at all.

I was asked, "What's best to do for this man now?" I commented she might acknowledge his sense of embarrassment. I went on to say there seems to be two implicit rules in this marriage, one that women should play a martyr role and another that men should work at tasks set by their wives; i.e., she has power, but must suffer for exercizing it. I said I thought that neither of these people knew how to increase their social power effectively. I might add that my interpretations were somehow not fully understood: the underlying concepts are not familiar to neophytes.

The Rules Structure for Identity

The battle in which male and female identity are now being tested is defined by certain rules. *He* takes it for granted his wife cares for the kitchen, kids, and church. He takes his sexual privilege with her as his due. He assumes she will be sexually faithful to him. He assumes he will father a family, "bring home the bacon," and provide "a home over their heads." The women challenge his assumption they will do housework and care for children. They demand equal pay for equal work and seek to eliminate sexist connotation in the English language such as the generic term "he." The least militant but perhaps most fundamental cry is "I want to be *interesting!*" As one woman said to me, "You can go to a party tonight and talk about your cases. Everyone will be fascinated. But if I talk about clearing a clogged drain, which was pretty interesting to me, I know I'll be an utter bore." She wants to be acknowledged as having noteworthy identity, not a self interchangeable with countless other brood marms.

The heightened militancy of women vis-à-vis men results in a continuous scuffle. Sexual skirmishes are only part of the warring. He scores himself a loser and feels confused: One man stopped opening the door for ladies only to get jambed by others who expected to go first. Another told me of the complaining of his wife who related how awkward she felt walking with a Vienese professor, for the good man's wife came trailing along behind carrying his coat. I recall flirting with a feminist black and being rebuffed, only to be chagrined to see my Polish physician friend in a Charles Boyer interplay with the same woman. As another woman explained, "Because you know her and are American, you can't get away with that male chauvinist stuff and neither could she allow herself to allow you to." A woman colleague laughingly described another situation: She had been nursing a feeling of "What-an-ineffectual-man-I-have-married." It seems her husband, an attorney, was struggling ineffectually to repair a broken pipe in the basement. She knew how to fix the pipe but preferred to let him suffer so she could gloat and feel superior and miserable. As she said, men have the idea they are always supposed to know what's going on and be in control. For some men such scuffles as I have listed lead to impotence, for others to affairs, and for others to a feeling of confusion and despair.

His potency is of course in question too at the office. If Jewish, he can perhaps complain more easily about being victimized, without experiencing inner horror of paranoid madness. Even when he is captain of some ship, the firm sensation of the tiller in hand has been dulled. Control has been assumed by committees and machines. The greatest sense of lost freedom and entrapment in the total work day is often experienced in the seat of his expensive auto hemmed in by countless other autos as he listens to the same unbelievable news report every five minutes.

The Loss

Identity derives from participating in the games of social concourse, from self-respect, and from being beloved. To return to William James, the men of whom we are speaking cannot now say, "This is the real me!" They are losers in the strife for self-respect. To be a successful "male chauvinist pig" requires an admiring audience. More specifically and intimately, it requires a wife who applauds domination, enjoys enacting helplessness, and either enjoys or feigns enjoyment of sexual congress on *his* terms. All that is lost. Depression ensues. As Laing remarks, the depression is the result of the loss of a partner in a game.

Paranoid feelings are close to depression. For many of these men merely talking to a therapist represents a further humiliation. It is a small step from feeling, "I am no good" to "they know I am no good." The men I know who have experienced a loss of identity in this battle are still outwardly appearing successful people. But they are hurting and angry. They do not know where to turn. They are embarrassed by the many successful challenges of male hideouts and power sites. If he complains to his fellows, many will look upon him as pathetic, as a castrate who has given up his male birthright or as a neurotic who has never laid claim to it. I heard reproaches of this sort in a "male consciousness raising group" not too many weeks ago. The self image valued by these old heroes is one of quiet strength. He would be a rock, an oak tree, a winner who never quits.

Therapeutic Intervention

What can the therapist do to enhance progress and engender hope? Is the doctor going to say, "This disease is outside my practice," or "There's nothing wrong with you" or will he prescribe some mind-numbing medication? First of all, the therapist had best have his own house in order. I heard a psychiatrist say a few weeks ago, "Something is wrong. I mimic the ghetto blacks where I'm consultant. My wife and her friends are in protest groups. It's fem lib., Black Power, Gay Lib. — Hell, I'm not in any protest group but all these people keep wanting from me." Another man, a successful psychoanalyst, complained of his practice, "It's like being nibbled to death by ducks."

A therapist might well begin by offering understanding: one interpretation of this male syndrome, which has a compelling effect, is the following, said with empathy: "Take me out, coach." This remark interprets the trouble in a particularly apt metaphor. This man feels grateful to be perceived as a fellow engaged in a tough life game, not wanting to quit, not wanting to admit being battered. He is marvelously understood by a doctor who can speak the words which he cannot. I heard another, similar therapeutic remark. It also spoke to the competitive struggle; it went like this: "He tight kept his lips compressed scarce any blood came through" (Robert Browning, "An Incident of the French Camp"). As a recipient of this remark explained to me, "It felt good to have the doctor understand what it is like to be a boy with your mouth bloodied from a fist fight. You're in the fight for honor, trying to look good to mom or dad or the coach and not really sure it all makes any sense but you know 'Big boys don't cry!' "

I do not maintain such interpretations were "curative" but they were temporarily liberating, allowing these men to feel better, more in touch with another human, more in awareness with their feelings. Each was more effective and less depressed for several weeks thereafter.

I especially like the poetic lines that evoke the "tight-lipped" image. It calls to mind Grant Wood's *American Gothic*. This middle-aged male is the grandson of those two severe farmers. At the same time, we owe our therapeutic expertise largely to the teachings of German psychoanalysts. The metaphors from their European experience are scholarly in reference, alluding to arts and letters and mythic symbols. I imagine those teachers to have been full-lipped, passionate, and even mystical. The content of their metaphors does not sit four square the imagery of soil, the weather report, the Sears Roebuck Catalogue, the New Testament, and mass transit. There is ample evidence for this conclusion; my own is drawn from years spent at Michigan and Pennsylvania, but you may easily infer the same from the attitudes of the White House. To approach this man, it is more helpful to understand locker-room slogans, such as, "A winner never quits and a quitter never wins," and "It is not whether you win or lose, but how you play the game."

Opportunities in Crisis

Therapists know something about "games" these days and how to enlighten the players. The term *game* is used many ways; generally it is an activity engaged in that has rules and some way to score the players. For young people, permission to play is "freedom," while for some older people, liberation is breaking the rules of the game. This middle-aged man of whom we are speaking conceives himself to be in some sort of big game and is convinced the other players are cheating. And yet he can discern no infraction so gross that he is willing to quit. Having been in a favored position, he is less able to perceive the erosion of liberty all about him and conceives his own losses as singular and shameful. By talking about it he can socialize his loss.[2] But we can do more. We can join forces and figure out how to survive and to savor that survival.

He may be reluctant to take a fresh perspective. I have talked to several men in their late sixties and seventies who are starting fresh businesses and fresh competitions with all their old gusto. That is the old game, the old rules, replayed. A new frame of rules can provide the base of a new identity. An art teacher's example was helpful to me.

This teacher was trying to help an evening class enjoy painting as an abstraction in colors arranged within a rectangular frame. He thinks the success of a painting depends upon whether the abstraction and colors work together and whether it pleases the maker and the viewer. He explained that the typical beginner seeks to compete with Rembrandt or Van Gogh. Even if he emulates these masters, the tyro will never get the pleasure of invention. But if the amateur painter can aim to please himself without imitating old masters, he has some chance of success. This particular painter, knowing the problem was his as much as any beginner's, began to run the colors of his paintings outside the frame and onto the walls of his home. As he explained to me, he exhausted the possibilities of working happily within the frame and decided to go outside. He was then able to integrate his painting a new way into his environment. We can generalize from this enlightening example. One can first endeavor to exhaust the possibilities of conventional life styles. When that no longer works, move out. How this example best applies to a particular case you will of course have to decide.

The issue of adultery and remarriage is frequent at our clinic. Appropos, it seems to be better to battle out the issues with the spouse, when the infidelity comes to light, than to part in coldness. Couples nowadays have the opportunity to thrash their difficulties out before a therapist rather than be forced by old rules into divorce and into greater identity fragmentation. Perhaps the greatest opportunity to the person over 40 is to take a fresh perspective on his identity. He can reassess his values, obligations, and responsibilities, and seek adventures under a new plume. After 40 one starts to reevaluate the game of marriage, the game of golf, the game of General Motors, and so forth. We are, to be sure, less able to reorient ourselves in regard to the earliest learned roles but can often back off from the competitive games of adolescence and young adulthood. We can go through a healthy process of disillusionment. The result is an opportunity to invest one's energy more by choice, to savor the passing moment rather than to be suspended in a conditional existence. For example, both husbands and wives ought to be able to share laughter in that cartoon in the *New Yorker* which portrayed a woman in her kitchen with youngsters hanging on her skirt saying, "I sweat all day over a hot stove while you're working in a nice cool sewer!" And older couples are harder to sell, a little more certain what hurts. In a cartoon showing a conference of cigarette advertizing men, one man shows a sign to the others on which is printed "Cancer is Good for You," and says, "How's this boss?" After forty, people ought to have the guts to look at what they consume and figure out what feels good even if it turns out to be old values such as hard work and thrift.

I used to hear the phrase, "Life begins at Forty." At age 20 I did not know what it meant; during my thirties I thought the phrase was merely a joke to deny the fear of growing old. Now, well past 40, I see that life does begin at 40. The rebirth of the middle-aged man in the crisis of confrontation with love and work is through reconsidering his life. This jump to a new perspective bridges the gap in historical continuity and establishes personal sameness in a changing world. The fresh sense of identity includes and heals what has been lost.

REFERENCES

1. Erikson, E. *Identity, Youth & Crisis*. Norton, 1967.
2. Burke, K. "Socialization of Loss" from "Dictionary of Pivotal Terms" in *Perspectives by Incongruity*.

Part II: Self, Salvation, and Psychotherapy

Preface to Part II: Self, Salvation, and Psychotherapy

ROBERT L. VOSBURG, M.D.

The notion of *self* in Western countries is uniquely individualistic. Perhaps all prehistorical cultures conceptualized each person as somehow special. Historically, the concept of self alludes to a physical self, a political self, and a spiritual self. Each self is governed by rules: the physical self by hungers, the political self by temporal emperors, and the spiritual self by god. Scholars attempt to codify the rules. The concept of *salvation* means to preserve some aspects of ourselves in the face of inevitable death. It has been a main task of religion to preserve the *spirit*. The preoccupations of modern psychology with emotion and cognition is a similar task conducted by sometimes different means. Psychotherapy is a modern attempt to abet the good, or godly, life. To understand *psychotherapy*, surely some comprehension of the older concepts of redemption and salvation is required.

The conventional meanings of *redemption* outlined by a collegiate dictionary are mercantile; to *redeem* is to buy back. Synonyms include *deliver, ransom, reclaim,* and *save. Redemption* implies releasing from bondage or penalties by giving what is demanded or necessary. A *redemptioner,* in the eighteenth and nineteenth centuries, was an immigrant who came to America paying for passage by becoming an indentured servant. *Saving* is a more general term conveying preserving. *Salvation* takes on sectarian nuances. Generally meaning the saving of man from the effects of sin, it conveys saving of the "mind" or "spirit" from the decaying flesh. Religions are often classified as being of two main types: one, "religions of attainment," in which man is expected to work out his salvation through his own disciplined spirit; the other, "religions of redemption," in which the diety is expected to take the initiative to save men and to prescribe the conditions of salvation. (Chamberlain, R. B. *The Dartmouth Bible*. Boston: Houghton Mifflin, 1961.)

Psychotherapy is an attempt to improve the subjective quality of the lives of human beings. As practiced in the Western world, it is an amalgam of old religious concepts and new psychological methods. The theme of the conference, "Self, Salvation, and Psychotherapy," recognizes this blend of old and new.

Which Self Does Psychotherapy Realize?

Irving Markowitz, M.D.

The concept that the sense of self is almost fully defined early in life with relatively limited possibilities of change is very attractive to psychotherapists. It allows therapists to draw sweeping diagnostic conclusions from meager data. It defines and limits involvement. It excuses failure. The working through of the transference becomes simpler the more totally the patient is considered to be "still back there" rather than "here." The concept that the sense of self is the continuing fluctuating product of every interaction has none of these advantages and is, therefore, considered less valid.

If we accept the extreme view that the individual sees himself *only* as others see him, we conceive of the self as a thermometer rising and falling with every change in outside climate. If we conceive of identity as fully established early in life, we see the individual as totally impervious to transient contact requiring the repetitive hammer blows of daily therapy to produce relatively minor changes. Neither of these extremes may be valid. To say that our role may make us does not imply that it will un-make us. To recognize that an individual may be very different as a mother than a wife, different as a friend than a co-worker, implies only a continuing process of fusion between what history has wrought and what is presently required. Identity is not created or destroyed by chameleon-like adaptability nor is it clarified by the refusal to be versatile. Those who are steady as a rock have been more universally admired than those who shift ground easily. The man for all seasons has been the man who recognized no change in season. Actors who maintain their distinctive trademarks, are generally more acclaimed than those who are totally immersed in their roles. We would, perhaps, not put so high a premium on constancy of image if it were more widely recognized that a sense of one fixed self is an impoverished sense of self.

Identity crises cannot be avoided by maintaining a constant picture
in one's mind as to the nature of one's identity, whether masculine or
feminine, young or old, patrician or plebeian. What may avert confusion is the knowledge that one is continuous in the passage from past
to present, from role to role, from situation to situation. If one is to
avoid disorientation or depersonalization, role change has to move at
the pace that one's brain switchboard can tolerate. Pathology in maintaining one's identity is the inability to maintain a continuity of conceptualization as conditions change. Often a patient feels that if he
approaches a new situation in a new way, he will somehow disinte-
grate in the process and will be unrecognizable to himself and to others. Few of us indeed are healthy enough to be capable of endless
adaptation without clinging to some fixed way by which we know ourselves and by which others may know us. Often specific mannerisms
serve as reassurance as to who we are. We hold and play with objects.
We stroke our beards. We readjust our postures in familiar rhythms.
We smooth or curl our hair. These characteristics are the trademarks
that cartoonists and caricaturists often utilize to depict who someone
is. These trademarks no more establish identity than do the numerous
identity cards that define who human beings are by listing their numbers, birth dates, birthplaces, physical characteristics, and parentage.
If there is any one thing that seems more crucial to establishing who
we are than anything else, it may lie in doggedly clinging to our personal philosophies in the hope that these will provide some stability
in the midst of flux. That personal philosophies are not crucial becomes
obvious when individuals become converts whether through religion or
through psychotherapy. The new disciples may continue to quote their
newly learned scripture more frequently than the old established disciples do, either to familiarize themselves with the new doctrine or
to convince themselves that the new philosophy is preferable to that
which they followed previously. The new philosophy does, however,
become integrated into their personalities, even though it may be dis-
gorged more readily than ideas that were acquired earlier.

A new sense of self is possible when the individual is thoroughly
disillusioned with the old self, when he becomes, through various
techniques, receptive to new information, or when he seeks to find
acceptance by a new parental figure, becoming in the process the kind
of person that he or she fancies that this noble figure could have sired.

The auspices under which we operate often make possible a different acceptance of ourselves. The young professional woman who felt it was immature of her to want to be cuddled, that she should not "regress" to such childlike levels of behavior, was accepting the interdiction by her therapist of such "immature" behavior. Yet, in an encounter group she allowed herself to cuddle quite easily. The illusion of a fresh start frequently permits the emergence of behavior that would have been intolerable in the old situation.

What we are is whatever has been part of our experiencing; what we are not has never been part of our experiencing. The ways in which we approach experience determine whether it becomes part of ourselves. To experience only through our previous conceptions and misconceptions entrenches the old familiar self. The Catholic adulterer who filters the joy or anguish of his adultery solely through his Catholic dogma is unable to sense himself differently.

Most of us are persuaded or hypnotized to make whatever changes we do make in our sense of selves by the influence of potent figures in our lives. Rare, indeed, are those who change through the complete unfettering of their sensations, perceptions, and judgment. If we are to be ever at peace with our different selves in any enduring way, liberation would seem to be a more likely route than role modeling. The spell of one witch or fairy is all too easily lifted by another. In spite of the professed interest of therapists in liberation, in practice they more often cast spells than they liberate. The more aggressive the therapist, the more of a role model he becomes. Passive aggressors are more effective than active aggressors. Whom should we follow, if not those who, in some occult way, pose the greatest threat to us.

The role that offers the most satisfaction or the fewest problems is the one we tend to adopt most exclusively. The doctor who never lies professionally but frequently does so socially is expressing his preference for the role that seems to guarantee his integrity. As he finds himself more and more uncomfortable in his other roles, he will introduce the mien of the physician into all of his activity. He will constantly diagnose and treat his parents, his wife, and his children. As long as involvement with them remains professional, he can afford to be truthful with them and with himself.

Some housewives, accepting the role that has been thrust upon them through the centuries, make too much of a virtue out of their necessity and immerse themselves in endless household activity. Whatever distaste they may have felt for their roles originally becomes lost in the poise, courage, and efficiency with which they put their heads on the blocks of their dishwashers, stoves, and vacuum cleaners.

Many individuals, rather than clinging to one particular role, exhibit a virtuosity that seems to be uncalled for in the particular circumstances. The rapidity with which they switch roles seems more related to haunting memories than to the realistic need for flexibility. Thus an individual speaking to a given sibling will find himself using a voice like that sibling's, totally different from the voice he uses customarily. Whatever need he originally had to compliment, cajole, mock, or pacify that particular sibling continues to motivate his current behavior.

Only by efficient evaluation of the advantage that one role has over another in any circumstance can either an impoverished role fixity or too rapid oscillation from role to role be avoided. Those who have to steal the mantle of their elders or would not be caught dead wearing any marks of another personality are insufficiently free to borrow what they need forthrightly or reject what they cannot use.

Disintegration of the personality may occur when aspects of the personality that the individual can tolerate only in one specific role threaten to impinge upon his other roles. The father who feels fatherly to his wife and husbandly to his daughter is able to behave in ways deemed appropriate by the society only if he recognizes that his behavior must be inappropriate to his ideation. If he can maintain the continuity of his eroticism and is not swept away by it, he may allow it to remain in the forefront of his awareness, where it may greatly enhance both these relationships.

Timorous individuals have to keep different roles completely compartmentalized. Loose boundaries between roles are for them impermissible. Romantic love is one thing, parental love another. Hyde is Hyde and Jekyll is Jekyll. Unless they demarcate each clearly, they do not know how to behave.

A few human beings totally compartmentalize their roles, use their versatility to show off rather than relate, and abandon any one role so rapidly that they have little opportunity to assess its lasting worth. They seem to be constantly auditioning for a series of parts for which there is no obvious demand.

An analyst had audiotaped his interview with a patient who in the course of the session did quick dissolves from Jenny to Jane to Janice. The three characters were caricatures of Freud's id, ego, and super-ego. (Theories of the geography of the mind have always seemed calculated to appeal more to our literary than our scientific selves.) To the two analysts listening to the tape, the three characters had no distinguishable relationship to one another. Their voices and ways of speaking were totally different. The listening analysts, both independently, decided that each character appeared not only as the result of inner release mechanisms but also in response to the therapist's cues. Particular expressions of dissatisfaction, whether grunts or words, produced an immediate presentation of a new self. The therapist was the prompter who was saying, "Now Jane, Now Jenny, Now Janice," and the patient preternaturally alert to any slight cue that something different from what she was doing was required, responded instantly with a total personality change. Her inability to restrict these quick changes to appropriate occasions prevented her from receiving the kind of approval that she thought this display of versatility deserved. She had perhaps, been so conditioned by blame-fixing parents that it had become necessary for her to have a large number of totally different facades that could be trotted out in rapid succession as each progressive characterization failed. Perhaps those patients who have to shift very quickly from role to role in response to any slight cue have had childhood experiences that convinced them that great calamity would befall them if they did not act totally in accord with what their parents expected of them. What these patients say then very quickly is: "Well, if that won't do, will this, or this, or this?"

In listening to Jenny, Jane, and Janice all three analysts found themselves liking Jenny (the id) best, perhaps because the patient, too, seemed to like herself best in that role. Yet, if the analysts were polled as to which character they would have most likely persuaded her to adopt as her mainstay role, they would probably all have settled on Jane (the ego). In a roundabout way this outcome brings us to the title of this paper and the goal of this discussion.

Like all merchants, psychotherapists soon learn that they will be less troubled by their customers if they peddle a product of consistent quality. Their patients will be less jealous of one another, less querulous about the treatment they receive, and more likely to pay their bills on time. A constant image becomes convenient for the therapist. The therapist may recognize that constancy and tedium often are synonymous. The succession of 45-minute sessions seated in the same chair, exhibiting the same geniality, with only brief coffee-less breaks to purge himself of the effects of the previous patient's ill humors may eventually become depressing. The rewards, however, are generally sufficient to compensate for the boredom. The therapist seldom recognizes that the role-model he presents may be pressuring the patient into a similar way of life, frequently adopted by but depressing to most mass-production workers. The patient pursuing a constant image is not likely to realize the rewards that accrue to the therapist.

In classical therapy the patient is not likely to become acquainted with the therapist in other than the beneficent Buddha role encountered in the office. If only he too could adopt this seemingly consistent equanimity, he too could attain the therapist's lofty indifference to stress. Perhaps the appeal of classical therapy to the wealthy is that only the wealthy can maintain this model of immunity to life's hardships.

Often the patient does discern quite accurately the array of selves that the therapist commands, which may constitute the most enduring therapy the patient ever receives. When the therapist does reveal, however reluctantly, his feelings and frailties, endeavoring at the same time not to trap the patient in those feelings, this may free the patient from the tyranny of constancy.

To differentiate one's self from the therapist's self is not a body differentiation but a differentiation of concepts and goals. Such differentiation is simpler if the therapist emphasizes that no one arbitrary ethic governs all contingencies, that different problems require different solutions, and that the therapist is more than *what* the patient sees. By trying to maintain one fixed self that will supposedly serve well in all of his or her connections the patient (like all multipurpose compromises) becomes unable to perform well anywhere.

The common human dilemmas cannot be resolved by one fixed stance. If we list some of these dilemmas as: whether to be free or bound, predictable or surprising, diffuse or intense, earnest or casual, devious or straightforward, involved or distant, it is obvious that one can take no mean position that will provide a fulfilling mix of life's satisfactions. To attain the greatest possible satisfactions, the individual must be capable of oscillating from one stance to another—to be predictable one moment and surprising the next, devious in one situation and straightforward in another, conforming to one requirement, rebellious to another. The range of oscillation is determined by the individual's ability to tolerate ambiguity, which in itself is a measure of health. Manninger defined mental health as the capacity for unlimited adaptation to a relatively unselected environment. A repertoire of roles makes such adaptation easier. Some individuals cannot tolerate too great a range of oscillation without dire consequences for their emotional health. The emphasis with them should perhaps be on increasing their range to what they can tolerate, rather than restricting their activity so that they are always safe.

The constant ideal that therapists have presented for their patients to emulate is the "genital" individual-involved, conforming, earnest, assertive, warm, responsible, properly potent, and performing. Because of the therapist's lack of humor and flexibility in presenting this ideal, often talking it to death, and because the patient models himself on how he sees this ideal personified by the therapist, all of the ideals become distorted. Involvement becomes duty, assertiveness becomes insistence on unearned prerogatives, conformity becomes self-righteousness, warmth becomes responsiveness, responsibility becomes stolidity, earnestness, obsessiveness, and sexuality loses impulsivity and creativity to become sterile and asensual.

The therapeutic relationship generally attempts to reduplicate the original conflicts in the hope of resolution of these conflicts. Often the resolution of these conflicts is as curt, arbitrary, and autocratic as the old resolution and, as a result, reduplicates not only the conflict but also its resolution that entrenches the old familiar self. In fact, since the patient is likely to see the therapist as a better god than the original authorities in his life, the trauma of separation may be greater than what was experienced in the original separation. The patient ends up feeling he missed the boat twice, the second miss producing more anguish than the first.

At times, too, therapy creates a stereotyped self by assuming that the patient's relationship is transferential to a relationship that, to the degree fancied by the therapist, never existed. Thus, a patient who never sought much approval from his original parents may, because of the therapist's assumption that all human beings need and seek such approval, be compelled to live through the seeking, the not getting, and the not needing the full approval of the therapist. Having for the first time experienced such feelings, the patient becomes as stereotyped as those human beings who did experience such feelings with their parents.

Currently, therapists are struggling more and more to help their patients develop a greater repertoire of selves. To avoid the hazard of the inappropriate emergence of the wrong self at the wrong time, they must help the patient acquire some capacity to compartmentalize without loss of the interrelationship of the different compartments. The patient must be free and must learn to be as aware of the feelings of others as of his own. If he does not become aware of what goes on in individuals of different backgrounds than his own, he will ignore the cues essential to plucking from his portfolio the role most appropriate to the immediate situation. Therapists cannot confine themselves to defining the different roles the patient has to play. They must also be eager, despite the lack of opportunity for full openness, to reveal some of the different roles they play, if they are to avoid enshrining the dubious values of a constant image.

The Family and the Self

Theodore Lidz, M.D.

Convened here in Boston at a time when we celebrate the 200th anniversary of the start of our nation's struggle for independence, it may be well to pause and realize that as we enter this last quarter of the twentieth century we are involved in a new revolution, which, though scarcely noticed as yet, may turn out to be more significant than the atomic revolution in which we have been caught up for the past quarter century. It is a revolution that concerns an axiom of our founding fathers—the truth they held to be self-evident, that "all men are created equal." In its simplest terms it is the belief that what a person becomes, or if you will—what self a person develops—depends greatly on how and where he is raised and that whether created equal or not, there is little opportunity for equality or little equal opportunity for persons who grow up in deprived social and economic backgrounds. Herein lies a reorientation that underlies some of our most serious dilemmas and threatens to overthrow much of our established way of life.

Paradoxically, at a time when the rights of the individual and the importance of individuality are being emphasized, the responsibility of the individual for his own welfare is denied. If a youth cannot qualify for college, he should not be refused admission and penalized further because he had attended poor schools and did not have educated parents. We hear that a jailed murderer is a political prisoner. No, he had not committed a political assassination; he is a political prisoner because the Establishment let him grow up in slums, deprived, embittered, and without opportunity for fulfilling work. Our system is all mixed-up, how can we say we have equal justice before the law when most of those whom our legal system punishes are victims of the injustices of our social system (Ryan, 1971).

We are caught in a serious dilemma—a moral and ethical dilemma—whose impact is no where greater than upon those of us who are best able to understand that the sources of failure lie in the setting in which the person had been raised and in his childhood experiences. Yet, we must understand that society also has its rights and needs for protection from those who are dangerous to others whether we deem them criminal or mentally ill.

The problem is inherent in theories of determinism and has troubled me for a long time. Every now and again, perhaps every two to three years when the confusions of our social system back me up against the wall, I take a trip to another country where the inhabitants have a very different way of regarding life. I do not have to travel far—just into my library and pick up a book that transports me into that imaginary nowhere of Samuel Butler—to *Erewhon*—with its most trenchant subtle criticism of Western civilization and satire of it. You will recall in that country because of their prescience that people would become the slaves of machines—just as we indeed have become enslaved to the nuclear missile and our computerized assembly lines—they abolished machines and inventions. You may also recall that in Erewhon we find the first conceptualization of psychotherapists—they were called "straighteners"—engaged in treating criminals. In Erewhon, following Butler's determinist principles, criminals were treated and the sick were prosecuted and jailed. Butler, of course, recognized and wished to emphasize that criminals (in our terms) were no more responsible for their condition than persons with infectious diseases, and often far less dangerous. Well, in Erewhon I attended a trial along with Samuel Butler. The accused was a young man of 23 who despite a number of previous warnings by the courts and even several mild sentences for bronchitis, persisted in his criminal ways and now had developed a clear case of chronic tuberculosis. I wish to quote an excerpt from the speech the judge made in sentencing him to life imprisonment at hard labor:

You may say that it is not your fault. The answer is ready enough at hand, and it amounts to this—that if you had been born of healthy and well-to-do parents, and been well taken care of when you were a child, you would never have offended against the laws of your country. If you tell me that you had no hand in your parentage and education, and that it is therefore unjust to lay these things to your charge, I answer that whether your being in consumption is your fault or no, it is a fault in you, and it is my duty to see that against such faults as this the commonwealth shall be protected. You may say it is your misfortune to be a criminal, I answer that it is your crime to be unfortunate.

Satisfied with this solution or no, it is not illogical, and perhaps the most useful outcome of my talk will be to encourage those of you who have not been there, to spend some time in Erewhon, and those who have been to return from time to time, for it helps free us from the arbitrary stereotypes of thinking of our own culture.

If we wish to establish a more meaningful democracy with equality of opportunity for all, the response required of us as our nation enters its third century may seem clear. We must struggle to eliminate poverty, abolish the slums, institute racial equality without segregation, and equalize our school systems. We must bake all our bread of one dough and hope that it will not be utterly tasteless.

But when we pause and consider, we ask if such measures will suffice. Will they provide equality of opportunity? Do they confront the crucial issues? Of course, social and economic deprivation can stultify development; but does the youth fail to qualify for college because of the poor inner city secondary school alone, or because he grew up in a home without any books, or was it, perhaps, because his father opposed his mother's ambitions for her son? Is the man a murderer because he grew up deprived and embittered about his environment and opportunities or was it because of a lasting hatred planted within him by a brutal father who was but a transient visitor in the home for several years and then abandoned his wife and children? The problems are often inseparable and it is difficult to know whether the social and economic deprivation, the cultural deprivation, the emotional deprivation, or the emotional turmoil is most significant. In any event, we know that, on the one hand, cultural and emotional deprivations are not necessary concomitants of poverty and that, on the other, they are all too common among the well-to-do. What will happen to this child raised in the affluent suburb whose mother imbibes Bloody Marys before breakfast, lunch, and supper, and who resents the child's very being because he keeps her from her career or from her bridge club? What will happen to this boy who rarely sees his awesome father and whose mother cannot let him move out of the home to play with other children because she too is neglected by her husband, a man who is busy amassing a fortune to gain power that is rewarded by high prestige even when the money and power are achieved by crippling compulsivity or by white-collar criminality?

What I am saying, as an introduction to my topic "The Family and Self," is that the pursuit of our democratic ideal has landed us in a quandary. The Jeffersonian concept of assuring the future of the republic by universal education does not suffice. In order to provide a child with a reasonably equal opportunity in our contemporary world, he requires a family background with parents who are as capable as any of transmitting to him the knowledge and techniques of our culture, and who also provide him with a stable emotional environment in which he can thrive rather than be thwarted and blocked. It becomes apparent that although, as in all living organisms, genetic factors play a role and limit the extent of the equality with which we are born, environmental factors also play an obvious and very significant role. It took the settling of the New World—and particularly the United States, Canada, and Australia—where children were no longer so tied to the occupation, education, and social status of their parents to realize how greatly persons are shaped by their environments. It is no accident that instrumental, pluralistic philosophies of education developed in the United States where it became apparent, and even taken for granted, that children can be very different from their parents. Then Freud and Adolf Meyer opened the way for us to realize how greatly emotional difficulties that can so severely limit a person depend on how he is raised. It took careful observation and study to recognize how substantially a person's intelligence depends upon environmental stimulation, on the type of linguistic tools he acquires, and on not being blocked by emotional difficulties that prevent learning. Now we have become increasingly aware of how importantly what a person becomes depends on the family environment in which he is reared, and not primarily on the family "blood" or genes he inherits.

Now, we are rounding the circle and we begin to understand that socioeconomic deprivation often derives from emotional deprivation. Many of the serious frustrations of antipoverty programs are due to the failure to appreciate that two different groups exist in the lowest socioeconomic categories. One group comprises persons who have not yet had the opportunity to emerge from a state of poverty, largely the most recent impoverished arrivals in the cities and the rural dispossessed; the other group derives from families that declined into poverty because of the emotional instabilities and inadequate child-rearing of one or more prior generations. Indeed, most in Class V (Hollingshead and Redlich, 1958) are apt to be the offspring of persons who had been unable to provide them with the essential adaptive techniques of the culture, and who, in essence, raise children without a self, without an identity. Here in Boston, Malone, Pavenstedt, and their coworkers, have in their book *The Drifters* documented how the children from such families, mostly white, seem by the time they reach nursery school already doomed to a life of inadequacy and incompetence. Despite a pseudo-precocity, they were markedly delayed in perceptual development; their language was impoverished; their inability to generalize from one experience to another was striking. Impulsivity and inability to delay gratification were obvious; though careless about injuring themselves, they could be almost paralyzed by anxiety. They were distrustful of adults, and because they did not differentiate between most adults, it was difficult for teachers to establish a meaningful relationship with them. Minuchin et al. (1967) who studied families, mostly black and Puerto Rican, in New York with two or more children who were in trouble with the law found that all of these families were seriously disorganized, incapable of providing emotional security and the essentials of family life to their offspring. The parents experienced in their own childhoods little in their backgrounds to foster maturity, had inadequate models for identification, and showed marked learning defects themselves. In Pavenstedt's words, the parents had brought to their families of procreation "all the deprivations, dangers springing from uncontrolled impulses, excesses leading to aggressive and asocial acting out, inconsistencies of every sort" (Pavenstedt, 1967, p. 249). The households lacked routines, and the training and care of the children were markedly erratic. The parents seemed to lack that minimal requirement for child-rearing—the realization that "children are undifferentiated, impulsive beings who have to be nursed and coerced into differentiated growth" (Pavenstedt, 1967, p. 313). Thomas Cottle in his recent book, *A Family Album: Portraits of Intimacy and Kinship* (1974) provides haunting life tales of how disorganized homes give rise to disorganized lives.

Such families that give rise to anomic and deviant offspring are not limited to the urban slums and are even encountered among the well-to-do who manage to float for one or two generations on inherited wealth or in those who have found their wealth through connections with organized crime. In any event, the disorganized family whether in the inner city or on the margin of a rural town presents a serious challenge, for economic aid and even educational opportunity are unlikely to help these families or their offspring appreciably, and more far-reaching measures are required to halt the perpetuation of such individuals and families from generation to generation. In contrast, economic aid may well prevent many impoverished newcomers from falling into the group.

How do we go about promoting greater equality of opportunity? Let us not be unrealistic and seek to provide equal opportunity rather than, for the time being, seek to overcome the serious inequities due to social and economic deprivation and the emotional disturbances that permanently stunt, stultify, and embitter the next generation. Among the foremost measures required is a dominant concern for the integrity of the family at a time when many claim that the family is an outmoded failure, the source of most social and psychological ills, when some call for its abolition and promote various substitutes for it without knowing whether they are viable or not, and usually without being aware of the many essential tasks the family performs. Indeed, there are reasons to doubt that any other institution can adequately replace the family, and to believe that the disintegration of the family will be synonymous with the disintegration of our society. Rather than discard the family before we know what we are doing and risk the potentially devastating consequences of such changes, it would seem more sensible to study what the family is all about and why it may not be filling its functions effectively at the present time (Lidz, 1963).

We cannot solve problems until we have isolated them; my thesis is that the family is essential to the emergence of a competent self, and if we focus on learning why it is essential and how it functions, we may be able to foster the emotional security required to provide some semblance of equal opportunity for our children's children.

The approach that I promulgate holds that the childrearing techniques we have promoted have so often failed because of basic misconceptions in our theories of personality development. We have placed the primary emphasis on what should be done with the child, to the child, and for the child—the child's need for love and how he should be held, fed, bowel trained, weaned, talked to, and so forth. These are all significant matters but they neglect the much more important matter of the family setting in which they take place. Perhaps we have taken the family for granted because it is ubiquitous, and thus we have failed to appreciate how many vital functions it carries out.

Now, in examining "The Family and the Self," it seems necessary to consider the nature of the self, a word that can be defined in many different ways and that can be taken to mean one's personality, one's identity, perhaps one's ego identity, or simply the essential qualities of a person. In some psychoanalytic conceptualizations, the self includes the id, ego, and superego, whereas others consider the self a content of the mental apparatus that is contrasted with object representations (Kohut, 1971, pp. xiii–xvi). However, the "self" has a special connotation that the philosopher-sociologist George Henry Mead (1934) has elucidated. The self has a reflexive connotation as we find in the words "myself," "yourself," "herself." It underlines that unique human characteristic of being able to regard the self as an object. It is, so to speak, composed of a "me" as well as an "I." It connotes the ability to be the perceived as well as the perceiver, the evaluated as well as the evaluator, and, in particular, the guided as well as the guide. It conveys that a person is able to grasp who he is and where he is, and thereby decide where he wants to go and to find a way to get there. As Mead noted, this ability to have a self—perhaps I should say to be a self—depends not only on the ability to use language and to think but also on the related fact that we are social beings. We gain the concept of ourselves through seeing other persons' selves as well as by our ability to consider how others regard us, react to us, and evaluate us, and thereby become able to regard and evaluate ourselves much as we consider others. Mead emphasized the importance of peer groups, particularly the peer groups of childhood, and of society as a whole to the establishment of a person's self-concept.

I believe, however, that Mead failed to appreciate how greatly the self—this reflexive self—takes form within the family. The child starts life undifferentiated from the mother and gains a sense of self as boundaries are established between the mother and the child. Then, how a child regards himself reflects how he believes his parents relate to him and regard him, giving rise to a self-evaluation that forms the foundation of how he will relate to others and how they will relate to him. To some extent his first name becomes the signifier of how members of his family regard him and relate to him in contrast to how they relate to others: he is Tom, not Bill, and certainly not Sue. Further, as he identifies with each of his parents or, if you will, internalizes them, his self-concept will also reflect his feelings about each of these parents and also each of his parent's attitudes toward the other. Because of such identifications or internalizations, the self also reflects an identification with his family as an entity because everyone assimilates ways that are more or less idiosyncratic to the family. To those outside the family he is a Ryan, a Johanson, or a Cohen and has an identity as part of a particular family and, as the names I have chosen indicate, this identity as a family member may often also contain elements of an ethnic heritage as well as the ethos of his specific family.

Herein lies an essential part of the revolution that I have been discussing—how much the development of the self depends upon the family in which the child matures. It is something of which we are aware but also something that we really do not wish to acknowledge. If we recognized how greatly the child's development depends upon the family environment, we are burdened with an awesome responsibility that may be more than we can bear. We are willing to accept the importance of genetic influences, for if we have conveyed them to our children, there is nothing we can do about it; we are even willing to accept the need for good nurturant care of the baby. Yes, we like to believe that natural childbirth, rooming-in, breast feeding, establishing a proper mutuality during the baby's infancy, proper bowel training, and so forth will assure the everlasting emotional health of the child. Should the child become a juvenile delinquent, an adolescent schizophrenic, or a drug addict it is because the pediatrician did not instruct the mother how to feed the baby correctly, or because the mother was depressed or simply ignorant and did not provide sufficient nurturant care those many years ago; nothing much can be done except to place him or her in the hands of a psychiatrist to try to undo the years of progressive maladjustment that ensued from the faulty handling by the mother when the child was an infant. Such views, perhaps more accepted by psychiatrists and psychoanalysts than by laymen, are an unbelievable oversimplification that defies common sense and, even more, what should be obvious to any psychiatrist not blinded by preconceptions or by the authority of his teachers.

Let us consider a moment. Here is a 15-year-old girl, Betsy, admitted to a psychiatric hospital, depressed and suicidal and perhaps somewhat paranoid. She has been ingesting methedrine in massive amounts as well as a variety of other drugs; because she has been afraid to sleep alone, her mother has let her boyfriend sleep with her each night and share the drugs that her brother procured for them. Yes, it is true that her mother was depressed when she was born, discouraged by the marital friction since the birth of their first child; it is also a fact that the mother had not provided satisfactory nurturance to the patient in the first year of her life. However, do we neglect the knowledge that the father had been unable to tolerate the attention the children required from his wife, began to drink heavily, and left the family when the patient was 8? Or that soon thereafter her mother started a series of affairs and when she became pregnant obtained a divorce in order to marry, only to find that her paramour was already married? Or that even though the father was extremely wealthy, the mother and children lived verging on poverty because of the poor divorce settlement the mother had been obliged to accept because of her extramarital pregnancy? Or what do we do with the sense of inadequacy conveyed by the mother who was unable to manage without the support of a man but was unable to hold a husband, or obtain a new one? How to explain that she had an adolescent lover live in the home when the patient was thirteen, or that she needed to confide her concerns about her failure to achieve orgasm to her 12-year-old daughter? Do we neglect the father's reluctance to support the patient and later his refusal to pay for her hospitalization? Or the mother's heavy use of tranquilizers? If these few items plucked from the family setting seem unusual to anyone, they have not had much experience with the families of adolescent girls who are addicted and compulsively act out sexually, unable to tolerate the overwhelming emptiness of being alone. If, however, one considers all the above as just an indication that the family consisted of sociopaths, let us consider for a moment a fragment of the life circumstances of a brilliant college student who suffered an acute but serious schizophrenic break during her second year at college. When she was 12, her mother, who always had seemed devoted to her and upon whom she had always been extremely dependent, suddenly disappeared. Not until weeks later did the mother write that she had run off with her hairdresser whom she intended to marry. The patient's stricken father then began to spend evenings in bars drinking, taking his daughter along to keep him company and listen to him berate her mother for deserting them. Then when she was 14 he took her on an extended trip abroad and, to save money, they slept in the same room often registered as man and wife.

The point I am trying to make is that almost all theories of child development have markedly oversimplified the process. A child does not gain an integrated self, a workable personality, simply through the proper nurturing of his inborn potential and being fortunate enough to escape from undue emotional trauma in early childhood, but rather requires positive direction, delimitation, and guidance from those who rear him in a family, or in some carefully contrived substitute for it. Attempts to study the child's personality development or maldevelopment without considering the family matrix in which it occurs distorts as much as it simplifies, and it is bound to error, for such abstractions eliminate the essentials in the process. The complexity of the molding influences exerted by the family have largely been overlooked because they are everywhere built into the functions of the family that, even when unaware of it, is responsible for fostering the child's development by carrying out a number of interrelated functions. I can give only an impression of these functions by categorizing them under several headings and through indicating what these headings include.

As the parental nurturant function has been well recognized, I shall here only mention that proper nurturance requires parents to have the capacities, knowledge, and empathy to alter their ways of relating to the child in accord with the child's changing needs. Also, the child's nurturant needs continue long past the oedipal period and include meeting the offspring's requirements for direction and delimitation well into adolescence.

What sort of nurture did Betsy receive? We cannot re-create the first year or two of her life, but we know that her mother was depressed and irritable during Betsy's infancy and the home was frequently disturbed by violent fights between her parents. Then her mother was preoccupied by two subsequent irritable children. When Betsy was 8—and when attachment to her father should be replacing her attachment to her mother—her father left the family, and her mother again became depressed. Then, the mother failed to be nurturant in the sense of setting limits upon the young adolescent girl.

We are aware that the structure of the self, in the sense of its division into what we designate as id, ego, and superego, is affected by parental behavior. As the superego is largely taken over from the parents—by their dictates but also by the internalization of their behavior—it follows that which id impulsions can be permitted direct expression, which can only find indirect expression, and which must be deeply repressed depend greatly on parental teachings and behavior. Well, Betsy, long before reaching adolescence, learned from her mother that a woman could use sex to attract someone to care for her, and that sleeping with various men was a proper earthy way of life— and much more. Further, as I have elaborated elsewhere, the integration of the child's self bears a very direct relationship to the dynamic structure of the family in which he is raised. The spouses' abilities to form a coalition as parents, to maintain boundaries between the generations, and to adhere to their respective gender roles are extremely important influences upon their children.

There was no parental coalition in Betsy's family, but rather, two immature parents who needed narcissistic gratification from the other and were constantly at odds about their children. The boundaries between generations were badly breached because the father behaved as a rival for the mother with the children, and resented the expectation that he be a parent; and then, the mother treated her pubertal daughter as a confidante, and sought her support and advice about her men friends. The parental gender roles were also confused, for the father stopped working at about the time Betsy was born and never held a job again, and he later refused to provide adequately for the family. Then, too, the family structure was disrupted because a child properly needs two parents, one of the same sex with whom to identify, and one of the opposite sex who becomes a basic love object, whose love can be gained by more or less identifying with the parent of the same sex. Here Betsy's oedipal transition was impaired because both parents constantly undercut the worth of the other; to be someone capable of winning father's love, Betsy needed to dis-identify rather than identify with her mother, and the father was not a suitable love object because Betsy's mother told her children that their father was sexually incompetent and probably homosexual.

The family also fills an essential function through being the first social system that the child knows and into which he grows. Here he gains familiarity with the basic roles as they are carried out in the society in which he lives: the roles of parents and child, of boy and girl, of man and woman, of husband and wife, etc. Within the family social system the child also learns about basic institutions and their values, such as the institutions of the family, marriage, and extended family systems. The motivation to participate in or to avoid participation in such institutions can be a major directive in personality development. It seems clear enough that Betsy gained a somewhat strange concept of mothers and fathers in her family, as well as of the advantages and disadvantages of marriage.

The family is also unknowingly largely responsible for enculturating its offspring. Most of the techniques of adaptation a person needs to survive are transmitted through the cultural heritage that is a filtrate of the collective experiences of his forebears. Aside from the actual techniques required for living in the physical and social environment, enculturation includes the mores and value systems of the society and, most important of all, the language, including its system of meanings and its logic that vary from one society to the other.

Returning to Betsy, we find that she gained a very flawed conception of the prescribed, permitted, and proscribed values of society from her mother and from the family transactions. I shall not here consider how her difficulties followed upon deficient confidence in the value of pursuing future rather than immediate gratification.

Another function of the family, which I have already mentioned, consists of providing the parental figures to serve the child as objects for identification. We say in the colloquial terms of psychiatry that much of the child's personality growth depends upon his internalization of parental objects. The identification with parents serves as the foundation for the development of the self. It is incorrect to think of these identifications only in terms of the relationships between a parent and the child, for much of the impetus to identify with a parent depends, as I have discussed, upon the affection and appreciation of that parent by his or her spouse. Betsy had little motive to identify with her mother who had been rejected by her father, and insofar as she identified with her mother she gained little if any strength to cope with problems, self-esteem, or a sense of being able to cope with a husband or children.

As we study the family's functions and how it carries them out, we begin to realize how serious the neglect of the influence of the family as a unit upon the child has been to our understanding of both personality development and psychopathology. We also appreciate that we have tended to overlook the obvious, namely, that who the parents are, how they behave, and how they relate to one another and what sort of family they create rather than the specific childrearing techniques they utilize are what may count most in the long run.

There is another aspect to the family's functions in the formation of the self. The self, I have been arguing, is, so to speak, shaped to a large degree in the family and by the family, but the development of the self in the sense of achieving an ego identity also involves the process of individuation. Psychoanalysis, largely due to the influence of Margaret Mahler (1971), has in recent years placed increasing emphasis on the process of separation-individuation, but its focus has been primarily on the early phases of the child's differentiation from the original symbiotic union with the mother. Various narcissistic disturbances have been attributed to the mother's failure to provide proper nurturance, particularly in terms of fostering proper boundary formation at the time when the child should be moving away from the symbiotic relationship. However, it is essential to realize that the child must differentiate not only from the mother but also from the family. The child differentiates from its family in two major steps: when it first leaves the nidus of the family to go to school during the so-called latency period, and when the adolescent prepares to form new cardinal and intimate relationships outside the family and also has the task of overcoming many of his intrapsychic bonds to family members and to the family as a unit (Blos, 1967). Paradoxically, the more solid the young child's emotional relatedness to the mother and the more fully the child's nurturant needs have been provided for, the more capable the child is to make an effective separation from the mother. Similarly, when the family carries out its essential childrearing tasks adequately, the child can differentiate from the family without too much anxiety and pain. When the family has provided the child the security of proper nurturance throughout the latency period and early adolescence, when the dynamic structure of the family has provided a scaffolding for the child's personality structure, when it has properly socialized and enculturated the offspring, and when the parents who have been internalized were themselves adequately self-sufficient, the child gains the foundations for becoming independent and for ultimately becoming interdependent with another. If we return to consider Betsy, one of the first things that becomes apparent is that she

was incapable of tolerating the anxieties of separation from her mother
in adolescence and immediately strove to form a new intense symbiotic or anaclitic relationship with a boy and sought to spend all of
her time with him. Sex, rather than a source of pleasure or the release of a drive, was a means of establishing a new dependency and
retaining the boy in a close relationship. When he was frightened by
her extreme possessiveness, she found that drugs could be a more reliable source of relief from anxiety than people. She had not been
provided with good nurturant care, a well-structured family, a workable set of mores, or a mother to internalize who was capable of being
a self-sufficient person, and so forth. In brief, although the problems
of the child's separation-individuation from the mother are basic and if
not accomplished adequately leave the person emotionally vulnerable
throughout life, it is also obvious that the process of separation from
the family is also of vital significance and that the ability to make an
adequate separation depends greatly upon how the family has filled its
various functions for the child during childhood and early adolescence.

Now what do these observations concerning the family and the self
have to do with our work in outpatient clinics or in mental health
centers? Currently many psychiatrists are in a phase of professional
discouragement, discouraged because of the minimal success of hastily
conceived mental health programs in achieving unrealistic goals—programs that often have become lost and diffused through lack of focus.
Now their relative failures—and they are failures only in relationship
to undue expectations—seem to be leading many to overemphasize again
the importance of hereditary factors, to magnify the occurrence of
"minimal brain damage," to await neurochemical explanations of
emotional disorders, to place most total reliance upon pharmacotherapy. They no longer wish to work with the complexities of a patient's
life experiences, a task for which they have received meager preparation in medical schools. After all, it is much easier to give drugs than
seek to modify the course of a life. We may well be moving to fulfill Huxley's satiric prediction in *Brave New World*—to a time when
people will be kept producing primarily to gain a weekend supply of
a drug that provides a synthetic escape and a transitory chemical
ecstasy.

I believe that recognition of the central importance of the family
unit can bring focus to our efforts in both prophylactic work and psy-

chotherapy. In our preventive efforts we can seek to diminish family shortcomings as childrearing agencies. We might, for example, focus more attention on marital counseling for, as I have indicated, the ability to rear children successfully depends greatly on the parental coalition. We might emphasize helping the parents with their insecurities as parents. We might take the Plunkett Society of New Zealand as an example, a voluntary agency that sends specially trained nurses into the home to make certain that the child is thriving and that the mother is familiar with and capable of carrying out adequate childrearing techniques. Every child born in New Zealand is visited at increasing intervals from birth until they enter kindergarten unless the parents decline such services. The Society also has special hospitals in which mother and infant are hospitalized if either the child or the mother fails to thrive during the child's first year of life. We might also follow the people of New Zealand in establishing throughout the country cooperative nursery schools in which the parents take turns caring for the children under the supervision of a skilled nursery school worker, and thus both help parents learn childrearing skills and also diminish the isolation of young mothers. We might seek men to fill some of the functions of surrogate fathers by being basketball and baseball coaches, cub scout leaders, etc. in inner cities where fatherless families are common. There are a wealth of such measures that can buttress the family and substitute for some shortcomings. Currently it may be most important to counter the growing tendency to inculcate the beliefs that the family is an outmoded institution, that one-parent families can function as well as intact families, and that communes devoid of family organization may be more satisfactory settings for rearing children. If we but grasp the importance of the functions of the family, we may move into a new era concerned not just with what a mother should do for and with her child, but rather with what the family as a unit need provide to foster the harmonious development of a child with a coherent and well-integrated self.

It may be useful to keep in mind what we have learned from the studies by Bradley Buell and his associates (1952), namely, that approximately 6 percent of the families in a city preempt about 45 percent of the health services and 55 percent of all the adjustment services including psychiatric service case work and protective supervision.

Thus, when we work with a catchment area, we may save considerable time and effort if, when possible, we look into the entire family situation and seek to foster improvements in the adjustment of the family as a unit. By focusing on these 6 percent of families as units, we may save enough time and effort to permit more work with patients with more favorable prognoses.

I am not advocating that the minimization of psychotherapy in favor of extensive social work nor that family therapy should replace individual psychotherapy. Indeed, it is particularly in individual therapy that we can gain focus by keeping in mind the central position of the patient's family in his development or maldevelopment and the importance of problems of separation and individuation from the family. Considerable confusion occurs in what we seek to do or achieve in psychotherapy. Are we focusing on making the unconscious conscious with a major intent of relieving the repression of drives? Are we following the dictum—where id was, there shall ego be? Are we seeking to permit the patient to express his hostility? Or to improve his sexual functioning? Is our primary purpose to improve his abilities to communicate and express himself? Many of these are reasonable goals; but, in a more general sense, we as psychotherapists have the creative task of listening to the patient's experiences, to the story he presents us with that has led to frustration, anxiety, and bitterness and that seems to be moving in the direction of an unhappy if not a tragic outcome, and, then, through examining it together with the patient help him begin to weave a less disastrous and, hopefully, a more satisfying way of life. Our goals vary with the situation, but in a general way, we seek to relieve underlying anxieties engendered by feelings of helplessness, and depressive symptoms stemming from hopelessness and open a path into the future for the patient. We recognize that in working with transference situations we are largely reexamining the patient's relationships with his parents to make it possible for his introjects of them no longer to interfere deleteriously with current and future relationships. We recognize that the patient's conflicting introjects, his transfer of fear or animosity, his misplaced erotic attractions, his confusions in gender identity, his needs for narcissistic gratifications, and much of the many other interferences to leading a reasonably satisfactory life derive from his experiences in his family of origin. Among the major reasons for psychotherapeutic failures is the failure to focus scrutiny on the personalities, relationships, and transactions in the patient's family of origin, and on the adequacies and inadequacies of the family milieu. We need not translate such matters into the esoteric terms of psychiatry—into terms of id, ego, and superego, or into levels of fixation, or oedipal rivalries if we do not have to mask our own confusions and ignorance. Indeed, when we work with a patient's life experiences in their own terms and when we seek to make them meaningful in terms of the patient's experiences with his parents and siblings, what we seek to do in psychotherapy becomes just as meaningful to the poorly educated and to patients from lower socioeconomic levels as to psychiatrists, clinical psychologists, social workers, graduate students, and their spouses, and those from the public relations industry who currently form the large majority of psychoanalytic patients.

In closing, I wish to return for a moment to the revolution that has been fostered by the realization that who a person becomes depends so greatly on how and where he is brought up, and particularly on the family of origin. As psychiatrists we are aware of the complexities involved and must not expect to reshape society within a generation. We can hope that by analyzing correctly the social problems that give rise to emotional disorders we can hasten the process of change through our mental health prophylactic efforts. As psychotherapists our job is primarily remedial. We hope by our efforts to help our patients overcome their blocks to self-expression and fulfillment and, even more, to live less embittered or futile lives. In so doing, we hope to make it possible for the next generation to have a better opportunity to realize their potential because of what we have done for their parents. We are aware that change takes time, but what we do of a remedial nature for this generation will be prophylactic for the next and permit its members to start life with a more equal opportunity than their parents. In a sense both we and our patients are in a position akin to many of our forebears who came to this country, perhaps with some meager hopes for themselves but often primarily in order to make it possible for their children to grow up in a new country with the freedom of its potentialities, a freedom that was in essence a release from the conditions that had frustrated generations of their ancestors.

REFERENCES

Blos, P. (1967). The Second Individuation Process of Adolescents. *Psychoanalytic Study of the Child,* 22: 162–86.

Buell, B. et al. (1952). *Community Planning for Human Services.* Columbia University Press, New York.

Cottle, T. J. (1974). *A Family Album: Portraits of Intimacy and Kinship.* New York: Harper & Row.

Hollingshead, A. and Redlich, F. C. (1958). *Social Class and Mental Illness.* New York: J. Wiley.

Huxley, A. (1932). *Brave New World.* New York: Harper & Row.

Kohut, H. (1971). *The Analysis of the Self.* New York: International Universities Press.

Lidz, T. (1963). *The Family and Human Adaptation.* New York: International Universities Press.

Mahler, M. (1971). A Study of the Separation-Individuation Process. *Psychoanalytic Study of the Child,* 26: 403–24.

Mead, G. H. (1934). *Mind, Self, and Society.* Chicago: University of Chicago Press.

Minuchin, S. et al. (1967). *Families of the Slums.* New York: Basic Books.

Parsons, T. and Bales, R. (1955). *Family, Socialization and Interaction Process.* Glencoe, Ill.: Free Press.

Pavenstedt, E., editor. (1967). *The Drifters: Children of Disorganized Lower-Class Families.* Boston: Little, Brown & Co.

Ryan, W. (1971). *Blaming the Victim.* New York: Pantheon Books.

Self-Image
in Pair Relationships

Etsuko Inselburg, M.A., M.S.W.

Definition of Self

Day in and day out, we, as clinicians, hear and talk about our patients in terms of their lack of self-esteem, lack of self-confidence, and poor self-image. We conclude from this talk that the way our patients feel towards self influences their way of life. Put another way, we can say that the way we perceive ourselves influences our behavior. People perceive the world in accordance with their ideas about themselves and, based upon that perception, they act. For example, Mary and John C. have been married for fifteen years. They consulted me when she was depressed. She reported that she felt inadequate. She met John when both were doing graduate work, but consequently she quit her studies to support John. Now John teaches at a college, and Mary cares for their three children, ages 14, 9, and 7. She chauffeurs kids to school and other activities and finds herself increasingly irritable and unhappy. Recently their 14-year-old son had a car accident. This event triggered the latest fight between Mary and John. Mary thinks she is an inadequate mother; furthermore she perceives her 14-year-old son David's accident as a *proof* of her inadequacy. Despite the fact that John attempted to console her and pointed out that the accident was outside her control, she persisted in feeling deficient.

At the same time we noted that John did not express shock or anger when he heard of the accident, despite his concern for the boy and investment in the automobile. It is my conviction that his benign reaction is best explained in terms of his need to maintain a self-image of ''gentle guy.''

Since 1920 in the United States, the concept of self has been the central issue among behavioral scientists whose approach is from the

"Symbolic Interaction" point of view.[1] However, no single or unified way exists to express this concept. The self has been variably referred to or inferred as "pure ego," "self-feeling," "reflected self," "ego," "phenomenal self," "self-esteem," "self-system," "ego-identity," "self-identity," "self-concept," and "self attitude." Differences among those expressions result from each author's point of emphasis. One emphasis is on self as a process or an aspect of "I." Another emphasis is on self as content or on aspect of "Me." Here "I" is an actor creating personal history moment to moment. "Me," on the other hand, is an object of observation and reflection by "I" a moment later. In other words, "I" appears experientially as a part of "me."

Though two aspects of the self, "I" and "Me," can be differentiated for the sake of clarification, it is impossible to distinguish in a daily life situation. They are two sides of one coin. For example, as soon as the person reflects, he passes from the experiential realm of "I" to the cognitive realm of "Me" and only clinical situations like group therapy enable us to observe the integration and discrepancy of "I" and "Me" (i.e., in the form of "peak experience" and "content-affect disjunction" respectively).

I will use the term self-image with an understanding that we are talking about a cognitive and affective attitude toward the self. There are at least three varieties of "self-image": the *present self,* meaning the way one sees himself as of now, expressed as "I am ———"; the *ideal self,* meaning the way one sees himself in terms of aspirations, expressed as "I ought to be ———"; and the *self-other self,* the way one imagines himself to appear in another's view, expressed as "I think my spouse sees me as ———." It is my objective to focus on the *present self* in this paper.

Once some idea about self has formed, it resists change.[2] Perceptions that threaten the self-image do not become clear. One persists in perceiving the old Gestalt. An unclear perception unfortunately produces "inadequate" behavior. Such behavior is unlikely to solve the tension and will likely contribute to the individual's feeling of being threatened.[3] In the case of Mary, to see herself as adequate entails a demand for responsibility that is too much for her to assume and act upon at that moment. So she persists in her inaccurate perception of herself, and of "the facts." For example, she feels that she played in the accident (i.e., she did not give David lunch on time) and therefore justifies her initial self-image as an inadequate mother. This perception does not help the feeling of being threatened but neither does it add to the threat by increasing the demand for personal competence.

Structure of Self-Image in Dyadic Relationship

When we think of ourselves in a given moment, that specific mental image must be drawn out of a larger picture, the whole configuration or Gestalt of one's self-image. Some aspects of self-image stand out as a figure, while other aspects remain as a ground.

For the past few years, I have been treating couples who sought help with disturbed marital and homosexual relationships. I decided to apply a test instrument that is designed to map out the *structure* of present self-image to this population.[4]

In my previous research, I devised "A Phenomenal Map of Self-Image" based on content analysis of 4,000 responses to the question "Who am I."[5] This map is divided in 18 different areas, according to time, space, and directional factors (see Figure 1). Our clients were asked to respond to this question "Who am I" and their responses were sorted out to make individual profiles (see Figure 2).

According to this method, our clients showed a striking similarity in one area, namely, absence of responses in the area #8, which is the present oriented, positive description of self in relation to one's significant others. The absence of statement in this area shows that our clients do not see themselves positively in relation to their significant others.[6]

Discussion of Self-Image in Dyadic Relationship

The absence of a positive self perception vis-à-vis significant others among our population might be explained away by saying "that's expected because these are the people who cannot get along with each other." But I thought a deeper explanation was required and began to examine the nature of pair relation in general terms.

Because I am Japanese, it is easy to perceive myself against different "others" or easy to perceive other Japanese against different "others." For instance, when I meet another Japanese here in the United States, the likelihood of forming a relationship with that Japanese is much higher than if we meet in Japan. When I spot a Japanese

THE PHENOMENAL MAP OF SELF IMAGE

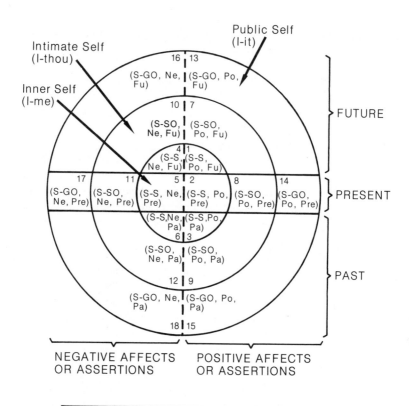

Figure 1

MARY B'S PHENOMENAL MAP OF SELF IMAGE

"Who Am I"   Statement

1. I have big knees
2. I feel unhappy
3. I depend too much on what other people think
4. I am a mother
5. I am getting old
6. I am married
7. I feel lonely
8. Friends make me feel I am inferior
9. I feel inadequate
10. I cannot deal with tension
11. I like to swim
12. I feel bored
13. I am trying to accept myself
14. I used to like to read
15. I don't have sense of direction
16. I like to lose weight
17. I am intelligent
18. I like to play bridge
19. I am honest
20. I don't understand my husband

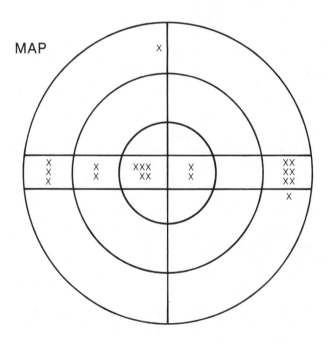

Figure 2

in the crowd I become alert and tense. I am dealing with the "Inclusion Anxiety." I send out feelers to determine whether I am adequate to him or he is adequate to me from the point of my self-image. In this example my sense of self worth is uppermost initially. I will be eager to be included by him if he appears to be attractive enough for me, so I make an effort to attract him as far as my self-image permits me to do so. Once I feel I am accepted, then I engage myself in negotiation with him in the area of power. Who is one-up or one-down will be decided at this stage. In the inclusion phase, we decide whether or not we will form a relation, while in the control phase we work out how we will relate. Whenever two people meet, these two stages occur. After he and I play out the drama of self-presentation, we may decide to be friends. We next begin negotiations about *sentiment* and *goal* in the relationship. "Sentiment" here is sum of our needs at different levels (biological, physiological, social, cultural, and existential) and affect attached to each need. "Goal" can be either a concrete or symbolic objective to which the direction of behavior is addressed.[7] When we discover we share common or similar goals, we not only feel comradely toward the partners, we strengthen our positive feelings toward each other by shouldering the part of the task derived from role differentiation in the process of achieving that goal.

Contrary to the idea so prevalent in general psychology, the *self* is neither a rock nor a persisting aggregation of traits. The *self* is a moment-to-moment perception of the actor. The significant other, usually the spouse (but not necessarily so), is one mirror. The other reflecting surface for self perception is what I call the "third element." This third element in the example of one Japanese meeting another is a perception of propriety (sensed as "we shouldn't get to know each other too rapidly"); the third element, however, can be anything in a given moment such as spouse's long working hours, neighbor's criticism, in-laws, spouse's ex-girlfriend, children, etc. The self-image in a pair relationship is defined by the phase of the relationship and the background—"third element"-"X." In this context any pair relation (dyad) is psychologically a triad because it always is influenced by this "X." Recognition of existence of "X," a recognition fostered by psychotherapy, is a threat to the pair because it causes a tension state. "X" demands the participants redefine the self-image for each in a triadic configuration.

Concluding Discussion of Self-Image Among Disturbed Dyads

In the example of Mary and John, Mary's perceptual field consists of herself (Mary) and other (John) and X (David) when Mary blamed herself for David's accident.

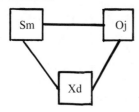

This triangle makes three sets of relationships from Mary's point of view, namely, Mary-John, Mary-David, John-David. For Mary to maintain a consistent perceptual field she must maintain a consistent self-image vis-à-vis John, David, and John-David. Thus, for Mary to be able to see herself as an adequate mother vis-à-vis David, the son, she has to see herself as an adequate wife vis-à-vis John, the husband. For Mary to be able to see herself as an adequate wife vis-à-vis John, the husband, she has to see herself as an adequate mother vis-à-vis David, the son. In both situations, she also has to be able to see herself as an adequate adult vis-à-vis John-David's pair. Moreover, for Mary to be able to see herself as an adequate mother, she has to be able to perceive David as an adequate son who needs her protection but with his own rights and John as an adequate husband who is involved with her but with his own rights too (see Figure 3).

As noted, what we do not perceive cannot threaten our self-image. Mary does not identify herself as an adequate mother primarily because she cannot acknowledge David as an independent young person with his own thoughts and feelings. Also her inability to see herself as an adequate wife who can carry a responsibility as a mature woman (i.e., with sexual intimacy) and inability to see John as an adequate husband with his own strength and weakness who cares for her contribute to her feelings of being an inadequate mother. David and John are perceived as either an impaired adult or an overgrown baby.

At the onset of an ordinary pair relationship, goals, mutual expectations, personal taboos, and childhood traumas are not spelled out clearly to the partner. The partners are not prepared to relate triadically. To ac-

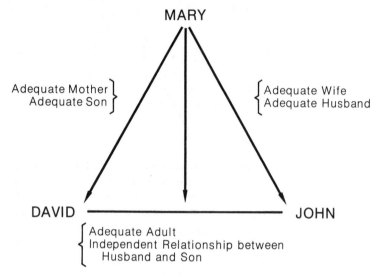

Figure 3

cept that one's partner lives in a different perceptual field that is constantly changing and is filled with different X's seems to be the key to the growth of both partnership and individual self in the relationship.

It is staggering for a therapist to observe how one partner ignores the complaints of the other. When people become used to each other, the other self melts in the background. Their appearance, voice, and actions evoke habitual responses. Mary did not hear John's consolation at the time of David's accident as a meaningful message to her. She just heard it as "John noises." When a couple loses the capacity to hear each other clearly, they have little choice other than living in private and distorted perceptual worlds.[8] Similarly, Mary was sure that John had thought of her as an inadequate mother for the past 15 years until one day in our office John said, "She is more than a good mother." I am sure John had said so many times in the past, but Mary could not hear. Now she realizes her real enemy is herself who thinks she "ought to be" a super mother.[9]

If you have followed my argument, you can now perceive that the absence of responses in #8 on our test has wide-reaching significance. The lack of statements that indicate a present-oriented positive description of self is not merely a reflection of being at odds with the partner but rather reflects a self-defensive expression stemming from the multiple expectations any person has of himself in a dyad such as marriage. The absence of responses in such a situation is due to a selective inattention to a painful aspect of the relationship between present self, significant other, and backdrop.

NOTES

1. "Symbolic Interaction" refers to the fact that human beings "interpret" or "define" each other's action and reaction. Response is based on "the meaning" of action and is mediated by "symbols." Herbert Blumer, "Society as Symbolic Interaction," *Human Behavior and Social Process,* ed. by Arnold M. Rose (Boston: Houghton Mifflin, 1962).

2. According to G. H. Mead, self consists of internalized attitudes and habitual conducts of significant others and generalized others. A child internalizes roles of parent, playmates, teammates, classmates, and the general public as he grows. By looking at himself through those people's eyes, his sense of self emerges and develops. G. H. Mead, *Mind, Self and Society* (Chicago: University of Chicago Press, 1934).

3. D. Snygg and A. W. Combs discuss the relation between Self Image and perception of the field in detail. Donald Snygg and A. W. Combs, *Individual Behavior* (New York: Harper, 1959).

4. My interest in this paper particularly lies in finding "Structure of Present Self-Image." Morris Rosenberg clarified the structure of Self Attitude and came up with eight different dimensions (content, direction, intensity, importance, salience, consistency, stability, and clarity). Then he focused on directional dimension and studied self-esteem. Though I appreciate his effort to get a sense of structure, if we go back to a component-study, we will lose interrelation of components, a sense of Gestalt. I prefer using an apperceptive test like TST. Morris Rosenberg, "Self Attitude and Other Attitudes," *Society and the Adolescent Self-Image* (Princeton: Princeton University Press, 1965).

5. "Who am I" question is called TST (Twenty Statement Test) and falls into the category of "apperception test." TST was originally formulated by Manford Kuhn to study "Self Attitude" of different religious group members. He asked the subject "Who am I" and checked the *number* and *order* of "consensual statement" among these twenty responses. I asked my sub-

ject the same question with Kuhn but treated the responses in a different way. Manford Kuhn and Thomas S. Partland, "An Empirical Investigation of Self Attitude." *American Sociological Review,* vol. 19, no. 1, 1954; Etsuko Sato, "Self Image," unpublished M.A. dissertation, St. Paul University-Tokyo, 1969.

6. Example of #8 responses:

Our Population	*Control Group*
"I am a daughter"	"I feel love from my family"
"I am lonely"	"Part of me feels I am nobody unless I have a man who loves me"
"I am a teacher"	"I enjoy working with children in my classroom"
"I have many friends"	"Among friends, I don't mind revealing myself"
"I am a mother"	"I am a mother of four children"

7. For "Sentiment" see Homans, "The Group and Mental Health," *The Human Group,* 1950. For "Goal," see T. Newcomb, "Motivation in Social Behavior," *Social Psychology* (London: Tavistock Publications, 1952).

8. We are talking about the discrepancy between Present-self-image and Self-other-image. The following authors made an effort to correlate marital disharmony with this discrepancy. R. D. Laing et al., "Disturbed and Nondisturbed Marriage," *Interpersonal Perception* (London: Tavistock Publications, 1966). Other studies are: R. F. Dymond, "Interpersonal Perception and Marital Happiness," *Canadian Journal of Psychology,* vol. 8, no. 3, 1954; E. B. Luckey, "Marital Satisfaction and Its Association with Congruence of Perception," *Marriage and Family Living,* vol. 22, 1960.

9. The example here is a triad in "I-Me" space (X being ideal self). The gap between Ideal Self Image and Present Self Image is one of the central issues by K. Horney to understand Neurosis. Karen Horney, *Out Inner Conflicts* (New York: W. W. Norton & Co., 1966). The studies in this area are: S. W. Caplan, "The Effect of Group Counseling in Junior High School Boys' Concept of Themselves in School," *Journal of Counseling Psychology,* vol. 4, 1957; R. F. Dymond, "Adjustment Changes Over Therapy From Self-Sorts," Rogers and Dymond (eds.), *Psychology and Personality Change* (Chicago: University of Chicago Press, 1954); C. R. Rogers, "Changes in the Maturity of Behavior as Related to Therapy," ibid; T. N. Ewing, "Changes in Attitude During Counseling," *Journal of Consulting Psychology,* vol. 1, 1954; I. Friedman, "Phenomenal, Ideal and Projected Conception of Self," *Journal of Abnormal and Social Psychology,* vol. 51, 1955; J. S. Hillson and P. Warchel, "Attitude Toward Self," *Journal of Educational Sociology,* vol. 30, 1957; H. R. Rogers, "The Self Concept in Paranoid Schizophrenia," *Journal of Clinical Psychology,* vol. 14, 1958.

The Place of Drugs
in Psychotherapy

Matthew J. Friedman, M.D.

There is great opposition to the use of drugs that affect the mind. People suffering from depression, anxiety, or schizophrenia often argue vehemently with the therapist who suggests that medication might help to alleviate their suffering. Members of the youth culture who wish to experiment with "mind expanding" drugs are under increasing pressure from their colleagues to seek "natural highs" rather than "highs" induced artificially. Finally and perhaps most surprisingly of all, intense opposition exists on the part of a multitude of psychotherapists who regard the prescribing of a psychoactive drug as either second-rate therapy or as a sign of failure.

What makes this attitude especially interesting is that there is very little disagreement about the efficacy of drugs themselves. Few people question the potency of antidepressants, anxiolytics, tranquilizers, analgesics, or hallucinogens. The arguments begin when a decision has to be made whether or not a psychoactive drug *should* be taken. In this regard psychiatry is in a very different situation than her sister medical specialties. Pneumonia *must* be treated with antibiotics. Heart failure *must* be treated with digitalis. There are no value judgments in these decisions, no conflicting therapeutic models to weigh against each other. Why then do many psychiatrists hesitate before prescribing an antidepressant for a patient with a classic endogenous depression? Why do psychologists, psychiatric nurses, and social workers hesitate even longer before requesting that their clients be evaluated for pharmacological treatment?

R. D. Laing has defined psychotherapy as "an obstinate attempt of two people to recover the wholeness of being human through the relationship between them."[1] This is an inspiring description of our work and a goal to which many of us aspire. How can a person become a "whole human being" if he is taking some artificial chemical that affects his mind? To become whole is to become free of psychotic terrors or neurotic anxiety. To become whole is to achieve the full potential of the Self, unfettered by unconscious constraints or situational concerns. In short, this approach sees psychotherapy as a search for the Self as it can be and should be. Therefore, drug therapy must be opposed vigorously because the drug itself becomes another obstacle to overcome before the Self can become whole.

Is there any evidence that drugs actually do interfere with psychotherapy? According to a very recent monograph by the Group for the Advancement of Psychiatry the answer is clearly "No!"[2] There is absolutely no systematic evidence that psychoactive drugs, appropriately prescribed, interfere with the psychotherapy of schizophrenia, depression, or neuroses. In the therapy of schizophrenia, insight psychotherapy by itself is of dubious value whereas treatment with major tranquilizers is essential. In the therapy of depression, pharmacotherapy and psychotherapy clearly complement one another: drugs elevate mood and reduce relapse rates while psychotherapy improves communication skills and interpersonal relationships. In the treatment of neurotic anxiety the issue is less clearcut and will be discussed at length below. Suffice to say that the question is not whether drugs can alleviate anxiety (because they surely can) but whether the therapist *ought* to administer such drugs to the anxious patient undergoing psychotherapy.

Thus we possess numerous effective drugs for a variety of psychiatric problems but in some circles it is considered wrong to resort to such pharmacotherapy. Likewise, it is considered wrong to receive blood transfusions by certain religious groups even when it is the only method by which life might be prolonged. The decision not to accept a blood transfusion is a moral not a scientific or medical decision. In such a case adherence to religious values has a much higher priority than life itself. In similar fashion, the abhorrence of drugs that flourishes among many psychotherapists is based either on a concept of therapy that fears serious consequences from drugs or that considers pharmacotherapy as somehow immoral. According to this view, taking a drug is a "crutch." Insight psychotherapy is "first class" treatment and the patient who needs a drug is a "second class patient." Gerald Klerman has labeled this attitude "Pharmacological

Calvinism.'' In a passage that anticipates the theme of this conference, Klerman writes:

In psychiatry we believe that secular redemption comes only through psychotherapy—insight is the secular equivalent of salvation through faith. If an individual uses a psychoactive drug, he is apologetic about it. . . . if you deal with your problems by yourselves, with will power, you are somehow more saintly than those who need ''drugs'' as crutches.[3]

Pharmacological Calvinism

Most Americans are opposed to the use of psychoactive drugs. Such opposition is not based on a concept of psychotherapy that equates insight with salvation but rather is based on an attitude towards mental illness itself. Several years ago a nationwide survey of attitudes towards drug use was conducted in which 40 percent of the respondents agreed with the statement that ''One of the main causes of mental illness is lack of moral strength or will.''[4] Thus there is serious question in the minds of many Americans about the legitimacy of psychiatric problems and whether ''mental illness'' really is an ''illness.'' No wonder that 87 percent (of the 2,552 respondents) agreed that it was better to use will power to solve mental problems than to use minor tranquilizers. It is interesting to note that the strongest critics of drug use were those people who had never taken a psychotherapeutic drug. Even among the respondents who had previously taken minor tranquilizers, 30 percent agreed that to have accepted drug therapy was a sign of weakness, and 42 percent reported that minor tranquilizers prevent people from working out their problems for themselves.

Among physicians who prescribe psychoactive drugs there is increasing alarm at the rate at which more and more prescriptions are being written for psychotropic drugs. Such concern has mostly focused on the anxiolytic benzodiazepine class of drugs, especially diazepam (valium) and chloridiazepoxide (librium). Commentators have denounced the ''relaxed attitude towards abusable drugs'' by physicians who tend to overprescribe tranquilizers, stimulants, and analgesics. Recently, in an effort to reverse physician-induced drug dependence, an extensive propaganda campaign was directed both at physicians and patients at a North Dakota Indian Reservation.[5] After several months of propaganda, prescriptions for all minor tranquilizers were reduced by 33 percent (although it should be noted that there was essentially no reduction in prescriptions for diazepam). The authors of this study clearly assert that it is wrong to take (or prescribe) minor tranquilizers and that it is good to curb their usage.

These studies illustrate Pharmacological Calvinism from the points of view of patient and physician. From the patient's side, minor tranquilizers reduce anxiety but should be avoided; mental illness is a moral defect and infirmity of the will that should be treated with insight therapy and will power. Use the will and not a pill! From the physician's side, too many drugs are prescribed because it is easier to write prescriptions than to spend enough time to help each patient deal with life stress and overcome anxiety.

A Necessary Evil?

In the face of such widespread negativism towards the pharmacotherapy of anxiety, how can one explain the phenomenal increase in psychoactive drug use among Americans. In 1972 more than 200 million dollars was spent on 77 million outpatient prescriptions for benzodiazepines (two-thirds of which were for diazepam). Furthermore, between 1970 and 1972, 30–35 percent of all benzodiazepine prescriptions were for patients who had not received such drugs in the past.[6] While discussing this remarkable annual increment in benzodiazepine usage, one commentator observed "at this rate the arrival of the millennium would coincide with the total tranquilisation of America."[7] At present it appears that emotional illness has replaced pain as the most common problem for which prescriptions are written. It also appears that 97 percent of all practicing physicians are prescribing diazepam for the emotional illness of their patients.[8] Even if we assume that physicians are selecting the most appropriate drug available, we must ask why are so many patients complaining of emotional problems and why are so many prescriptions being written?

Despite the widespread belief that people overuse drugs and abuse minor tranquilizers that they receive from physicians, evidence indicates that patients actually do not abuse drugs that are prescribed for them. This point is illustrated by a study conducted on the psychiatric ward at the University of Cincinnati Medical Center where the minor tranquilizer, diazepam, was freely available to any patient who requested it.[9] With this experimental design the investigators were able to assess the drug-seeking behavior of patients and the probability that they would "get hooked" on diazepam. They found that one-quarter of the patients never requested diazepam and that the vast majority of patients used diazepam conservatively and only requested it for "an appropriate indication of anxiety."

We thus face a paradox. Despite a value system that embraces the stoicism implicit in Pharmacological Calvinism, vast numbers of Americans are taking minor tranquilizers furnished by the majority of practicing physicians. *The Three Penny Opera* by Bertold Brecht and Kurt Weill has a refrain: "first feed the face and then talk right or wrong." I suggest that the prevalence of minor tranquilizer usage in the United States indicates a need that is so basic that Americans will scuttle their values for the sake of necessary relief from the human condition as they know it. It is wrong to take pills but it is too painful not to seek relief from the tension, complexity, uncertainty, and impotent rage that one experiences in the present-day United States. Drugs thus become a necessary evil and the necessity easily outweighs the evil.

What does any of this paper have to do with the question of Drugs and the Self? The Pharmacological Calvinist believes that minor tranquilizers just cover up the real trouble and prevent people from working out their problems for themselves. Perhaps it is just the other way around. Perhaps by alleviating the mental anguish induced by biological, intrapsychic, or situational factors, drugs actually facilitate the search for Self.

Complementing Psychotherapy with Drugs

With regard to the Search for Self, the discussion thus far has focused on drugs as a means for alleviating suffering. The drug itself is seen as a tool by which the individual can regain normalcy. Insight, enlightenment, and salvation are not available in capsules or elixers. Such an approach to therapy sees the natural human state as one without pain, psychosis, depression, and anxiety. The psychiatrist who defines his goal as the alleviation of suffering and restoration of function is quite satisfied if medication has reversed a crisis and permitted his patient to return to a life *that the patient defines as satisfactory*. Such an approach is not at all apologetic about providing symptomatic relief. The somatic therapist takes his cue from the patient in a fashion quite consistent with traditional medical practice. The goal is pragmatic and neither therapist nor patient is concerned with personality change or self-actualization.

The issue is more complex for psychiatrists who attempt to complement insight psychotherapy with pharmacotherapy. Some psychiatrists have a neutral attitude towards drugs, regarding them neither harmful nor particularly beneficial. They prefer not to use drugs because they see little benefit in pharmacotherapy but they will not withhold medication when it is obviously indicated. A second group of psychiatrists believe that drugs can alleviate acute suffering and thereby enable the patient to participate more efficiently in insight therapy. And there is a third group of psychiatrists who believe that pharmacotherapy may significantly facilitate treatment by bolstering ego functions needed for successful therapeutic interaction; they are convinced that judicious administration of drugs may produce enhanced verbal skills, clearer cognitive functioning, improved memory, and better concentration. All of these three groups of psychiatrists, however, agree that the goal of therapy is personal growth and development through insight. The patient definitely desires more than symptomatic relief, and he does not wish to return to life as he has known it previously. The patient wishes to explore himself as he was, as he is, as he might have been, and as he might yet become. He hopes to discover the potential within that he now defines as Self. Therapy is a learning process for uncovering and actualizing Self in the present and future. Drugs can assist in this process but do not deserve major credit for whatever is accomplished in therapy. Drugs are merely props, sometimes necessary but never sufficient by themselves.

Straight vs. Stoned Thinking

And finally, there is the point of view that sees psychoactive drugs as crucial factors in the Search for Self. Drugs are regarded as potent agents that promote or heighten a sense of self-awareness and open doors to other realities. Therapists who employ psychodelic agents are in complete disagreement with Pharmacological Calvinists. They see the drug as a divine gift to be employed creatively by those who seek personal growth through insight.

The cataclysm produced by promoters of psychodelic drugs during the last decade has passed. But their experiences remain part of our cultural consciousness and the lure of adventure in inner space remains compelling. It is perhaps an irony of history that the scientifically synthesized drug, LSD, spearheaded the anti-scientific, anti-materialistic, cultural revolution of the sixties. Young people who found themselves unable to accept the external reality perceived by their senses, sought to discover subjective meaning through experimentation with psychodelic drugs. It was truly a search for Self as well as Salvation that evolved into the counterculture of the hippie era.

Timothy Leary, after an overwhelming psychodelic experience with mushrooms in 1960, reported that he had died and been reborn, that his psychodelic experience had produced a profound and positive change in his life. He urged others to do likewise. Leary and Alpert reported that 62 percent of 98 subjects who received psilocybin experienced insights, personality alterations, and positive life changes. Leary and Clark reported positive benefits from psychodelic drugs to inmates at the Massachusetts Correctional Institute.[10] In this therapeutic approach the drug and not the therapist was primarily responsible for insight or Self discovery. The therapist became an adjunct, a guide who helped interpret the psychodelic experience but who lacked power in his own right.

More contemporary practitioners of psychodelic therapy have attempted to make the psychodelic experience conform more with traditional approaches to psychotherapy. They argue that psychodelic drugs can accelerate therapy by making unconscious material more readily available to patient and therapist. Fantasy, abreaction, transference, memory recall, and psychic integration are all intensified during psychodelic therapy. The skilled therapist can help the patient incorporate this material and achieve a heightened sense of awareness that can be sustained indefinitely.[11]

Ironically enough, now that psychiatry slowly begins to evaluate psychodelic therapy, graduates of the drug culture are moving in another direction. Drugs are beginning to be placed in proper perspective as their glorification comes to an end. It is the altered state of conciousness that is emphasized, not the chemical agent by which it is produced. Drugs may enable an individual to transcend "Straight Thinking" and achieve the freedom of "Stoned Thinking." These phrases coined by Andrew Weil signify the pathway of psychic exploration. "Straight Thinking" is the world of the ego with its reliance on intellect, sensation, empiricism, and conscious process. "Stoned Thinking" is marked by "reliance on intuition as well as intellection," "acceptance of the ambivalent nature of things," and "experience of infinity in its positive aspect." In Weil's terms a trip to Stonesville is equivalent to exploring unconscious processes through psychotherapy. But the best way to alter consciousness is through Yoga and Buddhism, not through psychodelic drugs. "Natural highs" are much preferable to drug-induced "highs." In a statement very reminiscent of Pharmacological Calvinism, Weil cautions:

> Drugs do not hurt the body in the ways most physicians think; they do not hurt the mind in the ways most psychiatrists think; *but they can keep people from reaching the goal of consciousness developed to its highest potential* [italics mine] . . . at the very time that drugs are triggering valuable states of unconsciousness they are reinforcing the illusion that these states of consciousness arise from external reality rather than internal reality. Thus it is ironic that persons who have the most positive experiences with drugs may also be the ones who become most enmeshed in illusory ways of thinking about their own minds.[12]

Thus we have come full circle. Although Weil does not regard drugs as a necessary evil, he is in complete agreement with Pharmacological Calvinists that genuine insight can seldom be achieved through drugs.

Conclusions

We have reviewed a spectrum of attitudes: (1) Pharmacological Calvinism that abhors any use of psychoactive drugs, (2) somatic therapy that employs drugs pragmatically for relief of symptoms, (3) psychotherapy plus pharmacotherapy that regards drugs potentially helpful in achieving insight, (4) psychodelic psychotherapy that currently attempts to harness the effects of hallucinogens and channel them into more traditional therapeutic constructs, and (5) achieving an altered state of consciousness through meditation that regards drugs tolerantly but somewhat condescendingly. Clearly, there is little disagreement about the power of drugs. Insight cannot be achieved with a prescription. Even the most potent drugs cannot foster personal growth by themselves. The psychotherapist need not feel threatened by drugs, because they cannot replace him.

But drugs also have a proper place in psychiatry. The Pharmaco-logic Calvinists are wrong; mental illness is much more than a lack of moral strength or a weakness of the will. There is too much good genetic and biochemical evidence to ignore the biological aspects of schizophrenia and major affective illness. And it is inexcusable to withhold medication when pharmacotherapy is clearly indicated.

When a patient convincingly complains of pain, some physicians readily prescribe narcotic analgesics while others worry that the patient may become addicted to drugs. No one doubts that pain is present and no one doubts that narcotics will alleviate such pain. At issue is whether the pain *ought* to be reduced at the risk of future conse-quences. Similarly in psychiatry, we can usually agree that a patient is anxious or suffering from some inner turmoil, and we can usually agree that certain drugs will reduce this distress. At issue is whether it is therapeutically necessary for the patient to endure such discom-fort until he can resolve his problem.

I am not suggesting that all patients in psychotherapy should receive medication. I agree that too many physicians are prescribing too many minor tranquilizers, and I often find myself refusing or limiting pre-scriptions to patients with character disorders, situational reactions, or neurotic conflicts. However, when anxiety interferes with psycho-therapy or produces needless suffering, I believe that medication is indicated. In my experience, a problem that impels a patient to seek therapy is sufficient to keep him in therapy even when his anxiety has been reduced by drugs.

Pharmacological Calvinists believe it is good for the patient to re-main anxious for that motivates him to work in psychotherapy. That theoretical position is unsubstantiated by fact. In all studies on the interaction between drugs and psychotherapy in treating character disorders and neuroses, there is no evidence that patients receiving drugs show less progress in psychotherapy; the only question is whether medicated patients are more productive in therapy.[2] Thus, it remains an open question whether drugs facilitate psychotherapy of neuroses, but it is clear that they do not interfere with the therapeutic process.

There are no guidelines. The therapist must make choice based on his own attitude towards psychic discomfort and on his concept of therapy. For me the decision is simple. Since drugs do not hinder therapy and often provide considerable relief, I do not hesitate to prescribe medication when indicated. I am meeting the needs of my patients and in no way lowering my goals as a therapist. Nothing is mutually exclusive about insight and drugs except for the obstinate beliefs of certain people who practice psychotherapy.

REFERENCES

1. Laing, R. D. *The Politics of Experience*. New York: Ballantine Books, 1967, p. 53.

2. Group for the Advancement of Psychiatry. *Pharmacotherapy and Psychotherapy: Paradoxes, Problems and Progress*. Volume IX, Report no. 93. New York: Mental Health Materials Center, Inc., 1975.

3. Klerman, G. L. A Reaffirmation on the Efficacy of Psychoactive Drugs: A Response to Turner. *J. Drug Issues* 1: 312–19, 1971.

4. Manheimer, D. I., Davidson, S. T., Butler, M. B., Mellinger, G. D., Cisin, I. H., and Parry, H. J. Popular Attitudes and Beliefs About Tranquilizers. *Am. J. Psychiat.* 130: 1246–53, 1973.

5. Kaufman, A., Brickner, P. W., Varner, R., Mashburn, W. Tranquilizer Control. *J.A.M.A.* 221: 1504–06, 1972.

6. Greenblatt, D. J. and Shader, R. I. *Benzodiazepines in Clinical Practice*. New York: Raven Press, 1974.

7. Editorial. Benzodiazepines: Use, Overuse, Misuse, Abuse? *Lancet* 2: 1101–02, 1973.

8. Blackwell, B. Psychotropic Drugs in Use Today. *J.A.M.A.* 225: 1637–41, 1973.

9. Winstead, D. K., Anderson, A., Eilers, K., Blackwell, B., Zaremba, A. L. Diazepam on Demand. *Arch. Gen. Psychiat.* 30: 349–351, 1974.

10. Caldwell, W. V. *LSD Psychotherapy*. New York: Grove Press, 1968; these studies cited in Chapter 2.

11. Ibid; Chapter 6.

12. Weil, A. *The Natural Mind*. Boston: Houghton Mifflin Co., 1972, p. 72.

Child Language and an
Emerging Sense of Self

Carolyn Kessler, Ph.D.

Introduction

The emergence of language in the child is a portrait of the child's gradual resolution of the complex relationships between himself and the world around him. Involved is a profound process of differentiation, both in the acquisition of the structure of language and in the acquisition of a sense of self. Essentially the thesis of this paper is that child language and a sense of self share interrelationships reflecting something of each other.

What, if anything, can the child's early utterances such as *mommy sock, no milk, sweater chair, see hole?, her paint* tell us about the child's emerging sense of self? Neither theories of language acquisition nor theories of developmental psychology are as yet adequate to give us answers to this question. However, research in language development is providing an increasing amount of data to give a greater understanding of the language acquisition process. It is the purpose of this paper to look at some of that data, to relate it to a definition of language and a definition of sense of self, to see what glimpses the acquisition of various language processes and categories may give of the child's view of himself in relationships to his world. The specific structures to be examined include early two-word statements, negations, questions, grammatical functors such as prepositions and articles, inflections for tense and number, and, finally, subordinate and coordinate clause structures.

Definition of Language

Language is not easily defined. Sapir (1921, p. 8) identifies certain critical elements when he states: "Language is a purely human and non-instinctive method of communicating ideas, emotions, and desires by means of a system of voluntarily produced symbols.'' Current definitions of language amplify this definition by viewing language as rule-governed behavior, species-specific to man. In order to arrive at a closer understanding of the rules of language as distinguished from the behavior which utilizes them, transformational linguistics has drawn a distinction between language competence and language performance. Competence is the internalized set of rules available to the idealized speaker-hearer of a language; performance is the actual use of language. The internalized set of rules constitutes the grammar. Performance is constrained by the nature of those rules as well as many other factors, including memory, emotional states, and nonlinguistic variables.

Language, then, is essentially a communicative, social phenomenon. The user must operate within the code set by the conventions of the society to which that code belongs. Failure to apply the rules of the language is failure to communicate. If we observe the young child of approximately 18 months of age capable of combining two words into meaningful utterances, the communicative efficiency of that child is, at best, inefficient. But access to the rules of language and application of the strategies for its use are crucial for social integration.

What, then, does the gradual build-up of the rules of grammar, from two-word utterances to longer, more complex ones, tell us of the process of social integration of the young child? Clearly multidimensional developmental changes are involved.

Sense of Self

Slobin (1973) points out that the pacesetter in linguistic growth is the child's cognitive growth. In turn, cognitive growth is intimately connected with the developmental changes that ultimately result in a sense of self. These changes will involve the way the individual perceives, conceptualizes, thinks about reality.

If we consider Piaget's distinction between egocentric and socialized speech, we may be able to examine how the child's language development mirrors the development of a sense of self. As Piaget views egocentrism, the term does not mean preoccupation with self but, rather, a limited awareness of self in relationship to others. Initially, the child does not differentiate himself from the surrounding reality. He is, as Brown (1965, p. 220) summarizes, "captive within his own point of view, not aware of other points of view and so cannot assume another's point of view."

At this time the child does not experience himself experiencing. Egocentrism manifests itself in an inability to explain something to another, to take into account the viewpoint of the listener. According to Piaget, the young child does not use language primarily in its social function of communication. Instead, he uses it to think aloud, expecting no answers, often not caring whether anyone is listening.

As the child undergoes developmental changes, the shift away from egocentrism requires him to distance or separate himself from the environment. The child then begins to organize experience, to perceive his environment, to act on and react to it. Evidence of the gradual shift from egocentrism to differentiation shows itself in socialized speech, as Piaget terms it. The child begins to convey information, make requests, give commands, make negations, ask questions. Eventually, differentiation leads to an ability not only to stand apart from the environment but also to contemplate it perceptually in the present, the past, or the future. As Hayman (1965) points out, once a child begins to refer to himself as *I* rather than by the impersonal form of his own name, he has advanced significantly in self-definition. Without denying its validity, such evidence provides only a very limited look, however, at the interrelationship between linguistic development and self-definition. Pronouns such as *I, me, mine, you, her, him* are found in the very early stages of language acquisition. To account more profoundly, then, for the relationship between the child's gradual construction of the grammar of his language and the emergence of his sense of self, we need to look beyond the surface elements of particular words or sets of words. What we need is a theory that can interlock language development with cognitive development. Although such a theory is not yet available, we can get glimpses of this interrelationship from current models of language design.

Theoretical Perspectives on Language Acquisition

As Lenneberg (1967) emphasizes, there is no evidence that the adults surrounding the child are the causative agents that determine language acquisition in the child. In ways not understood cognitive mechanisms of categorization, interrelation, or transformation operate on linguistic data that come to the child. Through hypothesis-formation and hypothesis-testing, the child constructs rules accounting for his grammar. At first these rules have minimal approximation to those of the adult grammar but, little by little, more refined hypotheses are generated until the child does indeed encode the grammar of his native language. Figure 1 illustrates the process of moving from a linguistic data input to the grammar of the language as the output.

Input: Linguistic   →   Black   →   Output: Grammar
       Data   Box   of the Language

FIGURE 1. OVERVIEW OF THE LANGUAGE ACQUISITION PROCESS.

Not understood is precisely what does happen in the black box. How is the linguistic data processed by the brain so that the child can formulate and use the rules of his native language? This process is an unknown. Nevertheless, in broad outline we can take note of some of the processes that must take place as we examine a scheme of linguistic organization.

Language involves the expression of meaning through sound. Meaning finds its origin in the conceptualization of a situation. If we take the sentence as the linguistic structure illustrating the kinds of relationships that must be established in the black box, we observe that the sentence represents a certain conceptual structure manifested in the pronunciation of that sentence. To move from conceptual structure to phonetic manifestation, three subsystems of language are involved: semantic, syntactic, phonological. The semantic system involves, among other things, the choice of lexical items or words. The syntactic system provides the rules governing the arrangement or ordering of the lexical items. The phonological system sets down the parameters for the phonetic manifestation of the sentence, of the surface structure. Figure 2 summarizes this theory of language design.

CONCEPTUAL STRUCTURE
↓

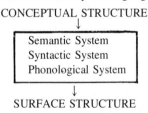

| Semantic System |
| Syntactic System |
| Phonological System |

↓
SURFACE STRUCTURE

FIGURE 2. OVERVIEW OF A THEORY OF LANGUAGE.

In order to acquire the rules of grammar, the child must be able to recognize the kinds of events that are encoded in language. And he must be able to process this information linguistically through all three subsystems of the language.

Until recently, it was generally assumed that the child acquires most of the grammar of his language by age 5. As linguists look more closely at Piaget's theory of cognitive development, this assumption is being challenged. Chomsky (1969) gives evidence that comprehension of some of the more exceptional patterns of English structure continues to develop through the period of age 5 to 10. Kessler (1971) and Tremaine (1975) found that bilingual children were still acquiring structures of their dominant native language well into the early school years. Ingram (1975) presents evidence that most of the transformational rules of English grammar are acquired between the ages of 6 and 12. Specifically, these findings show a remarkable correlation with Piaget's stages of cognitive development. Early language development correlates with the pre-operational stage defined by Piaget. Linguistic transformations of a complex nature appear in the stage of concrete operations as the child moves towards formal thought, the 6-to-12-year-old age range.

Specific Conceptual/Surface Structure Acquisitions

Brown (1973, p. 56) sets up five stages of language development based on the mean length of the utterance (MLU) as determined from the number of meaningful units or morphemes in the utterance. The MLU for Stage I begins at 1.75, for Stage II at 2.25, for Stage III at 2.75, for Stage IV at 3.50, for Stage V at 4.00.

To relate specific language acquisitions to the acquisition of a sense of self, let us take the child at Stage I. This stage is usually about 18 months of age. It should be possible, then, to look at linguistic structures in terms of the psychological or cognitive complexity of the notions they express. These notions, in turn, may provide us with clues to the strategy by which the child begins to differentiate himself from his environment. Specifically, we will examine some typical structures at the two-word stage. Following that, we will look at some semantic relations expressed in language: negation, questioning, spatial and temporal relations, definiteness, plurality. And finally, we will make brief reference to some of the complex operations of coordination and subordination of conceptual structures.

Two-Word Statements. Among transformational linguists who have attempted to define the semantics of the basic sentence relations are
Fillmore (1968, 1971) and Chafe (1970). Both are concerned with the
semantic roles noun phrases play in the conceptual structure proposition or sentence. Given the centrality of the verb, noun phrases associated with it may manifest a variety of semantic relations. A detailed
exposition of either Fillmore's or Chafe's model is beyond our purposes here, but it is pertinent to understanding the early stages of
language development to take note of certain semantic roles in particular. Among these roles are: agent, someone or something which
causes an action; object, the most semantically neutral relation; expe-
riencer, someone having a given experience; beneficiary, someone
who benefits from a state or process that may include possession; instrument, something used by an agent; location, the place of the action.

A study that examined some of these semantic intentions of child
language in its early stages is that of Bloom (1970). In demonstrating
the inadequacy of looking at the surface structure of children's utterances, she has shown that the context in which the child speaks is
crucial for revealing the underlying semantic relations. When a 21-
month-old child used *mommy sock* on two different occasions, the
contexts revealed quite different conceptual relations between *mommy*
and *sock* (Bloom, 1970, p. 5). In one case, it was in the situation of
mommy putting the child's sock on the child. Here the semantic roles
were those of agent-object. The other situation was that of the child
picking up her mother's sock. In that instance, the child was indicating possession-object relations in the statement *mommy sock*. When
the child said *sweater chair* while putting a sweater on a chair, the
underlying semantic roles were those of object-locative. Two-word
utterances indicate children have access to a wide range of semantic
roles.

Numerous examples of two-word utterances could be cited such as
eat cookie, dog jump, car big, that cat, kitty here, all of which indicate different underlying semantic relationships. What this example
illustrates is that from the earliest Stage I the child is using language
meaningfully. Furthermore, since language is, by definition, a social
phenomenon, the child uses it to communicate. Of significance, however, is the limitation of that ability to communicate. In early stages
of language acquisition, the child apparently can manipulate only two

and later three semantic roles at a time. This limitation places a heavy constraint on the child's ability to relate observations and events, a constraint on the differentiation of himself from his environment.

Negative Constructions. In studying the development of negative constructions in young children, Bloom (1970, p. 172 ff) distinguishes three categories of meaning: nonexistence, rejection, denial. In the child's earliest use of the negative *no* juxtaposed to a noun, Bloom found that the negative signaled nonexistence of an object. When a child could not find a pocket in the mother's skirt and said *no pocket,* the negation referred to the nonexistence of the pocket where there had been an expectation of its existence. One of Bloom's subjects used the negative syntactic devices *no more* to signal nonexistence of the reference such as in *no more juice, no more noise.*

The second category of negation to develop, as Bloom observed, is that of rejection in which the referent actually exists or is imminent within the contextual space of the speech event but is opposed or rejected by the child. When a child said *no dirty soap* as she pushed away a sliver of worn soap in favor of a new bar, the situation was no longer one of nonexistence but rather of rejection of something already present.

A third category in the order of development of negation is denial, distinguished on the basis of function rather than on structural devices. In denial the negative utterance asserts that a specific predication is not the case. The following situation illustrates denial in data collected by Bloom. The child asked *where's the truck,* referring to a toy truck. The mother picked up a toy car, handing it to the child as she said *there's the truck.* The child's response *no truck* denied the identity of the truck as car.

It is interesting to note that the same developmental order of negation contrasts has been reported for the native language acquisition of Japanese (McNeil and McNeil, 1968). Since one hypothesis about language acquisition is that it rests on a set of specific cognitive capacities, children acquiring language any place in the world impose the same features on language. These features appear as linguistic universals resulting from cognitive universals. It is also important to note that complex transformational operations are lacking in grammar of all three negation contrasts.

Development of negation may also suggest contrasts that gradually develop between the child and the environment. It would seem that reference to nonexistence of an object differentiates the child from his surroundings less than rejection of something already there. Denial goes further in indicating a capacity to stand apart from the environment. Denial manifests the ability to reject a predication, to oppose one predication against another. This ability would appear to be of considerably greater complexity than either a simple observation of the nonexistence of an object or rejection of a referent.

Question Formation. Another aspect of child language that may reveal something of the emerging sense of self is the ability to ask questions. English has two types of questions, *yes/no* questions, calling for a *yes* or *no* answer and the *wh*-question calling for some piece of information in the answer to *who, which, what, where, when, why.*

Children learn very early how to ask *yes/no* questions simply by changing the intonation to a rise at the end of utterances such as *no ear?* or *see hole?* This process avoids the more complex syntactic rules forming *do you see the hole?* Certain types of *wh*-questions also develop early. Ervin-Tripp (1970) states that in terms of production, *what* and *where* questions were both earliest to appear and most frequently used in her sample of children ranging in age from 1 year, 9 months (1,9) to 2 years, 5 months (2,5). By examining children's answers to *wh*-questions, Ervin-Tripp suggests an order of development with *what, where* followed by *whose, who, why, how,* and finally, *when.* The late acquisition of *when* questions undoubtedly is related to the late acquisition of a sense of time. Cromer (1968) found in his research on cognitive development that many time concepts do not develop until after age 4. Further attention to the acquisition of temporality will be given in the next section on modulation of meaning.

One characteristic of *wh*-questions in both Stage I and Stage II is that the *wh*-word is simply juxtaposed to a statement as in the example *what me think* or *why you smiling.* As observed for the negative structures, transformations necessary to produce the adult grammar questions *what do I think* or *why are you smiling* are absent.

Questioning, like negation, may also reflect the child's ability to distance himself from his environment. Simple *yes/no* questions undoubtedly reveal less differentiation than the use of *why* in asking for causality. This distance would seem to require considerable differentiation between self, the environment, and ability to manipulate and interrelate predications. Blank (1975), in studying the acquisition of *why* questions, found stages in which the child indicated acquisition of the meaning of *why* questions through the answers. During the first stage, the child may respond to a question such as *why is the dolly going to sleep* by ignoring the question, touching the dolly, or giving no response. Reasonable answers to *why* developed about age 3 in normal children. *Why* questions can place extraordinary demands on the child since often there is nothing in the situation to give the child a clue, either to giving a meaningful answer or in motivating the *why* question itself.

The gradual development of the ability to question, moving from *yes/no* types to the gradations of *wh*-questions may be an indicator of the development of an awareness of others and the conditions of surrounding reality, a moving away from the earlier lack of awareness of self in relationship to others.

Modulation of meaning. Modulation of meaning, as Brown (1973) uses the term, suggests a class of meaning that is in some ways less than essential. In particular, it is used to refer to markers needed to indicate verb tense, noun number, definiteness or lack of it, spatial or relational notions signaled by prepositions. Since these markers are somehow subordinate to the basic grammatical relations of a proposition, it is not surprising that they do not appear in a child's grammar until Stage II at the earliest, and in some cases, are not fully acquired even as late as Stage V.

In order of acquisition Brown (1973, p. 274) reports the following rank from earliest to latest acquisitions: (1) present progressive *-ing* suffix on verbs as *I going,* (2) prepositions *in* and *on,* (3) noun plurals as *two books,* (4) irregular past tense of verbs as *he ran,* (5) articles as *the/a book,* (6) regular past tense as *it snowed,* (7) present tense, third person of verbs as *he wants.* Semantically, this ordering encompasses several significant concepts: the notion of time expressed in verb present and past tense, the notion of number or plurality expressed in the noun suffix *-s*, the notion of spatial relations expressed in the prepositions *on* and *in*, the notion of definiteness in the distinction between articles such as *the* or *a*. Many of these modulations of meaning continue to be omitted even in school-age children, particularly under certain linguistic conditions.

Brown and others have tried to account for the observed ordering of these modulations of meaning in terms of grammatical or semantic complexity. Given the present limitations of linguistic models, there is yet no consensus on the right linguistic representations for rules governing these structures. Undoubtedly the ability to represent formally semantic concepts of temporality or plurality is linked to the cognitive development of the child. Possibly the notion of present tense, progressive aspect is less complex than that for past tense. Consequently, the child develops the -ing suffix on a verb well before the past tense -ed marker. Furthermore, spatial relationships manifested in prepositions on, in for locative case roles and the concept of plurality may also be less complex than the notion of definiteness expressed in articles as the/a. As Brown (1973, p. 369) notes, "there is no general theory of semantic complexity that makes it possible to assign complexity values . . ."

What may be significant, however, for the child's self-definition is the evidence that it is only as he moves into progressively more complex stages of language acquisition that recognition is made of plurality, or a range of spatial relations, definiteness, or temporal concepts. Not only are certain cognitive prerequisites necessary but also the child must be well beyond Piaget's stage of egocentrism. A kind of socialization or differentiation in which the child can take note of the present as differentiated from unseen past events, of more than one object differentiated from a whole, of a definite object as opposed to an amorphous group, of something above or below another all appear to reveal degrees in the acquisition of a self concept, a self concept that permits the child to separate himself from his environment and become aware of that differentiation.

Subordinate and Coordinate Clause Structures. Up to age 4 children's utterances are primarily simple sentences. In discourse, propositions are simply juxtaposed to each other. In describing a picture she had painted, a child age 3,6 gave this account:

That's a little bit of water. This is a whole gob of water.
That's a little bit. What is that funny noise? It talks.
This is about mommy and daddy. This is about a river.

Between ages 4 and 6 children begin to join propositions in a loosely connected way through extensive use of *and*. A boy age 4,8 described his painting made in the same Montessori class as the younger child cited above in the following connected set of propositions:

This is a ducks. And a tiger's coming. And there's the
tiger. I mean, there's the water floating on him. And
there's his feathers. And there's somebody sitting on it.
I mean, a bug and it's crawl on him and the bug's going to
eat him. This is a moving rock and it can talk. And it's
time to get out of the trap up here. The kid could kill it
and he was as big as the rock and he put it in the trap.
And see, it's a crossed trap and he can't get out of it.

Complex structures such as those making use of relative clauses are generally absent in the language of children below age 6. Relative clauses derive from transformations that subordinate one proposition to another. Also absent are complex coordinate structures such as those making use of *but, or, nor, either . . . or* and other such devices. In order to utilize the devices of subordination and coordination such as these, the child must be able to take the underlying conceptual structures of two or more propositions and interrelate them transformationally into a single structure. Ingram argues that most of the transformations of English are acquired between the ages of 6 and 12. A girl age 5,8, telling the story of her drawing in the same Montessori class as the previous two children begins to give evidence of this ability to operate transformationally on language structures. The following is the account of her drawing:

We're going to wear that in the summertime during Mark's birthday 'cause
he's only going to have a boy party and I'm going to have a girl party. You
know about Peter, my brother. And I don't know what he's going to do but
yesterday I was going to get my shoes to polish them and Peter was getting
his shoes to polish his and when I came back, he was polishing his.

This child gives evidence of just beginning to move beyond the stage of stringing propositions together with *and*, though she still uses it as a productive device. By this point, the use of *when* and *because* to introduce subordinate clauses as well as *but* to serve as a coordinator are part of her grammar. The resulting structures are products of transformational operations.

Piaget's theory of cognitive development predicts that complex transformations should develop in the concrete operational stage normally characteristic of children in the 6-to-12-year-old age range. At this point the child is capable of performing reversible operations. Such operations are reflected in the complex linguistic transformations relating one proposition with another.

Once the child has acquired the ability to operate on language transformationally, he stands in a new relationship to his language. He has a mastery or control that evidences profoundly integrated linguistic capacities. In terms of self-definition, the child linguistically capable of categorizing, subordinating, and relating through complex mechanisms more than one proposition is at a point at which he not only is clearly differentiated from his environment but also is, in turn, capable of acting on it.

Conclusion

In summary, we have looked at selected characteristics of the child's progression in language development from Stage I well beyond Stage V. We have examined some of the earliest two-word utterances, the process of acquiring negation and questioning, the refinements of meaning found in the expression of tense, number, prepositions, articles, and, finally, the formation of subordinate and coordinate structures relating two or more propositions. We have seen that each aspect of language development is in some way correlated with cognitive development. The pre-operational child cannot act on his language to the degree that the concrete operational child can when he performs complex transformations requiring reversible operations.

It is proposed that the progression in language acquisition reflects progression in the emergence of a sense of self. Just as the child gradually develops the ability to express certain conceptual structures, to act on them transformationally, he also gradually develops a sense of his own identity in relationship to or differentiated from his environment. Furthermore, it appears that the link between the emergence of self-concept and the acquisition of language is the degree of cognitive development. Figure 3 attempts to show this link, at the same time illustrating that the outer limits of all three—language development, cognitive development, self-concept development—are not well-defined.

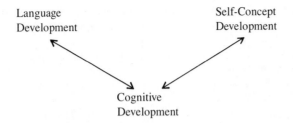

FIGURE 3. INTERRELATION OF DEVELOPMENT IN
LANGUAGE, COGNITION, AND SELF-CONCEPT.

Given the limitations in theories of language acquisition and cognitive development, any attempt to draw relationships must be considered exploratory and tentative. The unanswered questions remain
intriguing. Their resolution remains crucial to an understanding of
how the self comes to know himself.

REFERENCES

Blank, M. (1975). Mastering the Intangible through Language. Paper pre-
sented at the New York Academy of Science Symposium on Developmental
Psycholinguistics.
    Bloom, L. (1970). *Language Development: Form and Function in Emerging
Grammars*. Cambridge, Mass.: M.I.T. Press.
    Bowerman, M. (1973). *Early Syntactic Development*. Cambridge, England:
Cambridge University Press.
    Brown, R. (1965). *Social Psychology*. New York: The Free Press.
    ———. (1973). *A First Language: The Early Stages*. Cambridge, Mass.:
Harvard University Press.
    Chafe, W. (1970). *Meaning and the Structure of Language*. Chicago: Uni-
versity of Chicago Press.
    Chomsky, C. (1969). *The Acquisition of Syntax in Children from 5 to 10*.
Cambridge, Mass.: M.I.T. Press.
    Church, J. (1961). *Language and the Discovery of Reality*. New York: Ran-
dom House.
    Cromer, R. (1968). The Development of Temporal Reference during the
Acquisition of Language. Unpublished Ph.D. dissertation, Harvard University.
    de Villiers, J. and P. de Villiers. (1973). A Cross-sectional Study of the
Acquisition of Grammatical Morphemes in Child Speech. *Journal of Psycho-
linguistic Research* 2: 267–78.

Ervin-Tripp, S. (1970). Discourse Agreement: How Children Answer Questions. In *Cognition and the Development of Language*, J.R. Hayes (ed.), 79–107. New York: Wiley.

Fillmore, C. (1968). The Case for Case. In *Universals in Linguistic Theory*, E. Bach and R. Harms (eds.), 1–87. New York: Holt.

———. (1971). Some Problems for Case Grammar. *Georgetown University Monograph Series on Language and Linguistics* 24: 535–56.

Hayman, A. (1965). Verbalization and Identity. *International Journal of Psycho-Analysis* 46: 455–66.

Ingram, D. (1975). If and When Transformations are Acquired. Paper presented at the Georgetown University Round Table on Languages and Linguistics. To appear in Monograph series on language and linguistics. Washington, D.C.: Georgetown University Press.

Kessler, C. (1971). *The Acquisition of Syntax in Bilingual Children*. Washington, D.C.: Georgetown University Press.

Langacker, R. (1973). *Language and Its Structure*. New York: Harcourt, Brace, Jovanovich.

Lenneberg, R. (1967). *Biological Foundations of Language*. New York: Wiley.

McNeill, D. and N. B. McNeill. (1968). What Does a Child Mean When He Says 'No'? In *Proceedings of the conference on Language and Language Behavior*, E. Zale (ed.), 51–62. New York: Appleton-Century-Crofts.

Menyuk, P. (1971). *The Acquisition and Development of Language*. Englewood Cliffs, N.J.: Prentice-Hall.

Piaget, J. and B. Inhelder. (1969). *The Psychology of the Child*. London: Routledge & Kegan Paul.

Sapir, E. (1921). *Language*. New York: Harcourt Brace.

Slobin, D. (1973). Cognitive Prerequisites for the Development of Grammar. In *Studies of Child Language Development*, C. Ferguson and D. Slobin (eds.), 175–208. New York: Holt.

Tanz, C. (1974). Cognitive Principles Underlying Children's Errors in Pronominal Case-marking. *Journal of Child Language* 1: 271–76.

Tremaine, R. (1975). *Syntax and Piagetian Operational Thought*. Washington, D.C.: Georgetown University Press.

Wells, G. (1974). Learning to Code Experience through Language. *Journal of Child Language* 1: 243–69.

Psychotherapy and the Dilemma of the Death and Rebirth of the Self

Bernard J. Bergen, Ph.D.

It is clear that psychotherapy can no longer be regarded as a specialized form of medical or psychological treatment. In even the most general bookstores, books on every form of psychotherapy now stand next to analyses of social, economic, and political problems. There is an innate logic to this proximity. Although the disciplines that study human behavior differ in their methods and perspectives, in the final analysis they all address themselves to the common problem of human suffering. In its emergence as an important discipline in the Western World, psychotherapy has become a critical voice in the general discourse on the nature of human suffering that informs the ongoing history of ideas.

It has, I believe, become a critical voice because, in the decades since the end of Second World War, suffering has taken the form of what Erikson once termed, "a life style of patienthood" (1, p. 13). It is a term Erikson used, of course, to characterize young man Luther, and it refers to a "sense of imposed suffering, of an intense need for cure . . ." and in Kierkegaard's terms, "a passion for expressing and describing ones suffering" (1, p. 13). It is surely not accidental that Roth's *Portnoy's Complaint,* Vonnegut's *Breakfast of Champions,* and Heller's *Something's Happened* made the best-seller lists. They are not isolated phenomena but represent a dissection of suffering that pervades the novels, plays, films, and even, at times, television shows that reach all segments of society. People have become increasingly fascinated, in the most profound sense of that term, with catching a glimpse of their own suffering in images of suffering that are terribly familiar to therapists. The images of suffering in our time are variations of those images that leap out at us from between the dry clinical sentences of Freud's first case histories: images of persons whose presence in the world is an agony of speechlessness in the midst of what is called speech, an agony of falling away from what is real in the midst of what is called reality, an agony of experiencing a void in the midst of what is called the dense and the concrete. In the last few decades it is as if people have superimposed upon the traditional and even ancient socio-political and religious images of their suffering an image once thought not to be of this world: the madman. On the most commonplace streetcorners it is not unusual to hear people speak, in one way or another, the opening line of Ginsberg's *Howl:* "I saw the best minds of my generation destroyed by madness . . ." (2, p. 9).

Thus, whether or not it is true, as some have suggested, that all social and religious ideologies have exhausted themselves as guiding doctrines (3,4), it is certainly true that people are calling to psychotherapists to supply the answers to that double question posed by suffering: what is its nature? and what is the work to which it calls us? Psychotherapists, of course, have not been reluctant to answer this call. What they have offered as a response, I believe, has crystallized around what can be called the "theme of the death and rebirth of the self." As I see it, the somewhat awesome array of psychotherapies that have been invented in the last few decades represent, in one way or another, variations on that theme. This theme has emerged, however, in a more or less unreflective manner. It exists, I believe, as the largely unexamined standard by which psychotherapists measure what they can reasonably say in a discourse on human suffering.

The question I propose to raise, however, is whether or not the theme of the death and rebirth of the self poses a dilemma for psychotherapy which it must face more directly than it has yet done and which it must face now more than ever. I suggest that if it fails to do so, it will compromise the seriousness of what it offers people as a discourse through which they seek to answer the questions posed by their suffering. Before attempting to spell out this dilemma as I see it, let me try to clarify briefly what I mean by the theme of death and rebirth of the self.

Who is that person who comes to the psychotherapist complaining of suffering and to whom the psychotherapist speaks? On what horizon does he place that density of flesh and speech who sits before him so that he can grasp the meaning of that suffering? What psychotherapist today would not answer that it is the horizon of the socio-cultural world? Psychotherapists insist that they speak to a presence in the world who is a history within a prior history of culture. It is a self to whom they speak who was, in the beginning, only a potential that became a self through a history of being shaped and formed by its culture. In other words, there could be no self that speaks except as it was first spoken to; there could be no self except as it appears first on the ground of the speech of others who speak to it. But psychotherapists would also hold that the concept of an individual's history is not exhausted by a self which develops as the reflected speech of others. The full concept of the "history of a self" is held to be that of a history which points to the self's surpassing that of being the reflected speech of others in order to become a self which speaks for itself in its own right.

Erikson has given us one of the most influential concepts of this history of the self in his idea of the "struggle for identity." His concept of the "identity crisis" has made his work one of the most popular variations of the theme of death and rebirth of the self in the literature of psychotherapy. The "identity crisis" is his way of formulating the "moment" in the history of the self at which it intersects the history of its culture and engages in a struggle to surpass being a history it never made in order to become a maker of its own history. It is, Erikson tells us, "a critical period, a kind of second birth . . ." (1, p. 14). Erikson, I believe, clearly means for us to see the "identity crisis" not only as that which not only defines the developmental stages of adolescence and early youth, but also defines the enduring struggle that haunts everyman's life as it haunted, for example, the lives of those archetypal figures of suffering, Hamlet and Luther (1, 5, 6). He means for us to hear our own suffering in Luther's cry during his fit in the choir when he "roared with the voice of the bull . . . 'I am not' " (1, p. 23).

In other words, for Erikson, we are to understand our suffering as the sign of a self struggling to recover from experiencing itself as an affliction. Suffering is the struggle "to create something potentially new: a new person" (1, p. 20). We are to see ourselves like those patients who "want to be reborn in identity and to have another chance at becoming once-born, but this time on their own terms" (1, p. 103). But what is this struggle for rebirth actually about? Erikson gives us a glimpse of the vision that lies on the other side of the "death" of the afflicted self in the promise of the fulfillment of the life cycle stages of "intimacy," "generativity," and "integrity" (7). Abstracted from their theoretical grounding, they are a vision of what humans have longed for but have known only by their absence: love as fulfillment; work as meaningful; and, perhaps above all, to be able to die well, without rage and despair. At its heart, the rebirth of the self is a vision of the fulfillment of the self.

As I indicated, I am referring to Erikson in this badly abbreviated fashion, only to illustrate one variation on the theme of the death and rebirth of the self for the purpose of trying to clarify that theme. Needless to say, not all systems of psychotherapy ground themselves in the particulars of Erikson's theory of epigenetic stages and ego development. Yet, as I see it, almost all systems of psychotherapy enter a discourse on suffering with the idea that suffering is the self experiencing a terrible estrangement from itself that is a kind of death that calls to it to struggle to be reborn into fulfillment. And almost all systems of psychotherapy have at their heart the idea that this struggle of the self to be reborn into fulfillment is no less than a struggle to fulfill its fate.

I submit that this theme of the death and rebirth of the self poses a dilemma for psychotherapy. The dilemma exists because there are other voices that have entered the discourse on suffering that raise grave questions about believing in the possibility of a death and rebirth of the self. It is not that these voices are saying things that are particularly new, but that what they have to say has a compelling and urgent quality to it. The grave questions raised by these voices can be represented by a single play, Samuel Beckett's *Waiting for Godot*. First presented on the stage in 1955 when it was regarded as a somewhat "incomprehensible avant-garde work," it became only nine years later, an "all too easily understood modern classic . . ." (8, p. ix). In the absurd talk and actions of Vladimir and Estragon we are told that the possibility of a suffering self being reborn into a fulfillment of itself is an illusion. It is a belief in a cunning deceit that marks history, individual and social, as the history of a self-deception. The meaningfulness of that belief, its very possibility, is talk. Vladimir and Estragon give us talk as a circle that circles nothing, as words that are alien to the speaker at the moment he utters them to a listener who will not understand them. Talk is words that attempt to mobilize belief, but in the final analysis, we are told, what speaks and says everything are the silences and gaps between words—the absolute silences that answer the supplicant. Once born, we are being told, we are fated to die, and we cannot be reborn.

Beckett's play, however, points to more than a despairing nihilism. In staring down all beliefs it opens up a question that contains the very dilemma that confronts psychotherapy when it speaks about death and rebirth of the self. Vladimir and Estragon, waiting for the beginning of their journey toward fulfillment, wholeness, and completeness, commit a seemingly endless violence, both subtle and direct, on themselves and each other. The question which Beckett's play raises, and which is being raised by that myriad of voices that speak in a discourse on suffering in a manner similar to Beckett's, is this: Is it true that the desperation of human beings to give a density, substance, and concreteness to visions of rebirth of self is no less than the source of all violence?

I submit that Freud, for one, suggested this question in his work. If we abstract Freud's patients from the outdated language of instincts and psychic energies in which he entangles them, and even disregard the sometimes laborious interpretations he makes of their symptoms, they are given to us in his work in the ''pure'' image of the desperation to be reborn that represents a violence far from unfamiliar to us. His patients knew with certainty that their fulfillment was waiting for them ''out there.'' On the ground of this certainty, they established the meaning of their suffering as an affliction imposed on the self by something monstrous in the world that must be controlled, eliminated, made servile in the service of their rebirth.

Dora knew the reason for the affliction that was her life. It was her father. Did he not refuse to end his affair with his mistress? Did he not throw her into the clutches of a seducer? This is only part of the litany of crimes by which he betrayed her. There is no question but that her father is a selfish, unjust, and manipulating man. Freud does not seem surprised by this fact. The question for him is: what does Dora want from her father? Among other things, her symptom of aphonia, precipitated by her father's frequently absenting himself

from the house, tells us. As Freud put it: "When the person she loved
was away she gave up speaking; speech had lost its value since she
could not speak to *him*" (9, p. 50). When he left, she suffered a dying;
she wanted to be reborn. She wanted to render him into the servility
of the perfect lover who would give her a perfect love. What violence
on herself and on him would she not perform to reach this vision of
fulfillment? What violence have we not performed on ourselves and
others in the name of this vision of fulfillment?

The Wolf Man also knew the reason for his afflicted life. It appears
at the very beginning of the evolution of the complex structure of his
illness. "He began," Freud tells us, "to be cruel to small animals,
to catch flies and pull out their wings, to crush beetles underfoot; in
his imagination he liked beating large animals (horses) as well" (9,
p. 494). It was as if the flying, crawling, creeping, walking things
of the world surprised him by their freedom, and this surprise was
like a dying. They appeared in their freedom as monstrous evils that
imposed upon him a dreadful fault: the absence of power. In this
dream about the "six or seven" white wolves perched on a walnut tree
outside his bedroom window, the window, he told Freud, "opened of
its own accord" to let in the terrifying stare of the wolves (9, p. 498).
To end the defiling freedom of the things that populate the world by
commanding the powers of violence would purify his fault. What more
evidence of fulfillment is needed than the absolute immobilization of
nature's freedom? What violence would we not perform on nature to
reach this vision of fulfillment? The Elephant does not die because he
threatens the advancement of civilization—but to make billiard balls
and piano keys.

Schreber, the paranoid, also knew the reasons for his suffering.
His illness was a history of those reasons. First, his physician would
not give him the justice due him—to be a man (9, p. 398–99). Then
God Himself could not understand Schreber's agonizing struggle to
become a woman. God was flawed; He could not *see* the truth and
this flaw of blindness was a monstrous obstacle to be overcome if
Schreber and mankind were to be reborn into a perfect state (9, p.
404–05). And somewhere in all this the world itself becomes the
monster that imposes an affliction on his life. Schreber has a vision
of the end of the world in which "he himself was the only real man
surviving" (9, p. 455). Only "his ego was retained and the world

sacrificed . . . all things [had] become indifferent and irrelevant to him'' (9, p. 455–56).

Does Schreber mock us? His intertwined visions of violence and salvation are clearly paranoid delusions, the result of what Freud termed, ''the projection of an internal catastrophe'' (9, p. 457). But are we not living in a time when almost all things seem to have become indifferent and irrelevant to us? Ariés has said that in our time ''what is important is that one die in a manner that can be accepted and tolerated by the survivors'' (10, p. 7). He is speaking of a death resulting from ''natural causes.'' But it is only a small and easy step to apply his insight to human actions that cause death. Are we enraged at Lieutenant Calley because he committed murder or because he was indiscreet in doing it? Are we more shocked by his actions or his obvious stupidity? Are we furious at the plight of starving, diseased, and dying children who advertise that they want to be saved, or at their indiscretion for becoming visible? No matter how hard he dreamed, Schreber could not end the world; but our dreams are close to being filled with a density that would deny them as dreams.

Psychotherapy, I submit, cannot avoid the dilemma of reflecting on its own theme of the death and rebirth of the self as the possible source of all violence. In other words, it cannot avoid the dilemma of confronting its own voice within the general discourse on suffering, as a voice that may be speaking about dangerous illusions. It may well be a dangerous illusion to approach the self as if it were a moribund thing begging us to arouse it into the fulfillment that we envision as life. Do we populate history with an endless human bestiary—weasel kikes, bovine micks, gorilla niggers, slope head gooks—out of a rage born from a futile effort? Is the rebirth of the self an illusion we invent because we seek to run from the truth that once born there is no fate for the self but to die?

It is true that when psychotherapy poses these questions it confronts the dilemma of inflicting upon itself a narcissistic wound. It raises the spectre that as part of a discourse on suffering it may be contributing to a general sickness while masking as a cure. It faces the dilemma of being an important voice in a general discourse on suffering while not yet knowing what it is saying. To turn away from the dilemma, however, may mean paying the price of rendering itself silly and trivial. It does so, for example, when it declares, as did Greenacre, that ''most adults seem to accept their own identities without much contemplation . . .''

and only "young children, philosophers, artists and certain sick individuals concern themselves constantly with questions of their identities" (11, p. 148). Even the word "contemplation" and the demurrer "constantly" cannot save this situation from being an embarrassment in an American society whose members are preoccupied with establishing the "truth" of themselves as beleagured members of one or another kind of minority group.

Psychotherapy has come to play too important a role in a discourse on suffering to flee from that role by embracing silliness and trivia. Of all the disciplines that speak in a discourse on human suffering, psychotherapy above all knows that if truth is to be found, it is most likely to be found when those who speak have the courage to ask: "What am I saying?"

The author gratefully acknowledges the encouragement and suggestions of Dr. Robert Vosburg.

REFERENCES

1. Erik H. Erikson. *Young Man Luther*. W. W. Norton, (The Norton Library edition), 1962.
2. Allen Ginsberg. *Howl and Other Poems*. City Light Books, 1956.
3. Philip Rieff. *The Triumph of the Therapeutic*. Harper and Row, 1966.
4. Daniel Bell. *The End of Ideology*. Free Press, 1960.
5. Neil Friedman and Richard M. Jones. "On the Mutuality of the Oedipus Complex: Notes on the Hamlet Case" in M.D. Faber (ed.), *The Design Within*. Science House, 1970.
6. Erik H. Erikson. "Youth: Fidelity and Diversity," *Daedalus*. Winter 1962.
7. Erik H. Erikson. *Childhood and Society*. W. W. Norton, 1950.
8. Martin Esslin. *The Theatre of the Absurd*. Doubleday Anchor, 1969.
9. S. Freud. *Collected Papers*, vol. 3, Basic Books, 1959.
10. Phillipe Ariés. "Death Inside Out," *Hasting Center Studies*, 2: May 1974.
11. Quoted in Nathan Leites. *The New Ego*. Science House, 1971.